Trapeziometacarpal Joint Osteoarthritis

Simona Odella

Trapeziometacarpal Joint Osteoarthritis

Diagnosis and Treatment

Springer

Simona Odella
Istituto Ortopedico Gaetano Pini
Milan
Italy

ISBN 978-3-319-44334-8 ISBN 978-3-319-44336-2 (eBook)
https://doi.org/10.1007/978-3-319-44336-2

Library of Congress Control Number: 2018940446

Printed on acid-free paper

This Springer imprint is published by the registered company Springer International Publishing AG part of Springer Nature.
The registered company address is: Gewerbestrasse 11, 6330 Cham, Switzerland

Preface

Trapeziometacarpal arthritis is a common disease in female population over 50 years old. Thirty-two percent of people over the age of 50 years have radiological evidence of trapeziometacarpal joint osteoarthritis. In a population aged over 80 years, radiographic evidence of trapeziometacarpal osteoarthritis is as high as 91%, but despite a very high prevalence of radiographic osteoarthritis, particularly in the elderly population, the presence of radiological findings does not correlate well with symptoms. Often radiological advanced arthritis does not correlate with an important pain and functional limitation; instead initial radiological stages can be painful causing weakness and impairment in daily activities. It can happen that two persons with the same radiological findings may experience a high degree of pain and disability. As a result, trapeziometacarpal osteoarthritis is frequently treated based on symptoms rather than radiological investigation.

Conservative therapy is always the first choice. Only in case of failure and persistence of pain and dysfunction at the base of the thumb, surgery could be considered as a possible solution.

There are many different surgical procedures to treat thumb osteoarthritis: some of these are trapeziectomy with ligament reconstruction and tendon interposition (LRTI), trapeziectomy, trapeziectomy with ligament reconstruction, trapeziectomy with interpositional arthroplasty (IA), Artelon joint resurfacing, arthrodesis and Swanson joint replacement, partial trapeziectomy, partial trapeziectomy with pyrocarbon or PLDLA bioabsorbable interposition spacer, metacarpal osteotomy, and other different techniques.

In literature a systematic review has failed to identify any additional benefit in terms of pain, physical function, patient global assessment, strength, and adverse events of any procedure over another. There is no evidence that the shortening of the thumb, after simple trapezium excision, can cause pain or worse functional results [1].

The aim of this book is to give an overview of the anatomy of the thumb, the possible reasons that lead to the trapeziometacarpal joint degeneration and of the possible solution in case of thumb osteoarthritis, considering conservative treatments and surgical options; in both cases the aim is to decrease pain, increase strength, and improve physical function.

There is no evidence that a technique can give better results than another, and many different options have to be considered in any single case to give the correct indication. It is important to evaluate anatomical condition (trapezium bone stock, trapezium ipoplasia, joint instability), radiological stage, age of the patient, and functional demand before choosing the surgical technique.

Milan, Italy Simona Odella

Reference

1. Wajon A, Vinycomb T, Carr E, Edmunds I, Ada L (2015) Surgery for thumb (trapeziometacarpal joint) osteoarthritis. Cochrane Database Syst Rev (2):CD004631. https://doi.org/10.1002/14651858.CD004631.pub4

Contents

Anatomy of the Trapeziometacarpal Joint

1

One of the most important steps of human evolution is the development of a prehensile thumb.

In contrast to ape hand, whose thumb motion is limited only to flexion-extension movements [1], the human thumb also provides movements of opposition, retropulsion and circumduction due to the development of a biconcave-convex joint at the base of it: the trapeziometacarpal (TM) joint. The thumb is the only finger with polyaxial movement, and this turn enables us to grasp objects differing in shapes and sizes.

This feature makes possible fine motor skills and power grasp and gives the thumb a central role in hand function. In fact, loss of thumb function imparts a 40–50% impairment to upper extremity function [2].

The shape of the trapeziometacarpal joint is very different to the other carpometacarpal joints, and also the position in the space of the thumb is unique.

In fact, the axis of the thumb lies in a pronated position, flexed about 80° relative to the plane of the metacarpals of the fingers [3].

The TM joint is a biconcave-convex saddle joint (Fig. 1.1) that is characterized by a discrepancy of 34% of the articulating surfaces [4]; in fact the base of the first metacarpal is larger than the trapezial joint surface; the centre of rotation of trapeziometacarpal joint lies at its volar ulnar corner.

The discrepancy of articular surfaces and the laxity, in resting position without rotation, make possible a large range of movement, but adding the absence of bony constraint, it leads to an intrinsic instability of the joint; so, the stability of the TM joint relies only to several ligaments that stabilize the trapezium and the TM joint. The TMC joint is stable and tightly congruous with the home screw torque rotation phase in opposition; these unique multiplanar motions permit power grip, power pinch and delicate precision pinch.

The carpal trapezium articulates with the thumb metacarpal, index metacarpal, scaphoid and trapezoid; if there is a large medial osteophyte from the volar trapezium, it could interpose between index and thumb metacarpal.

S. Odella, *Trapeziometacarpal Joint Osteoarthritis*,
https://doi.org/10.1007/978-3-319-44336-2_1

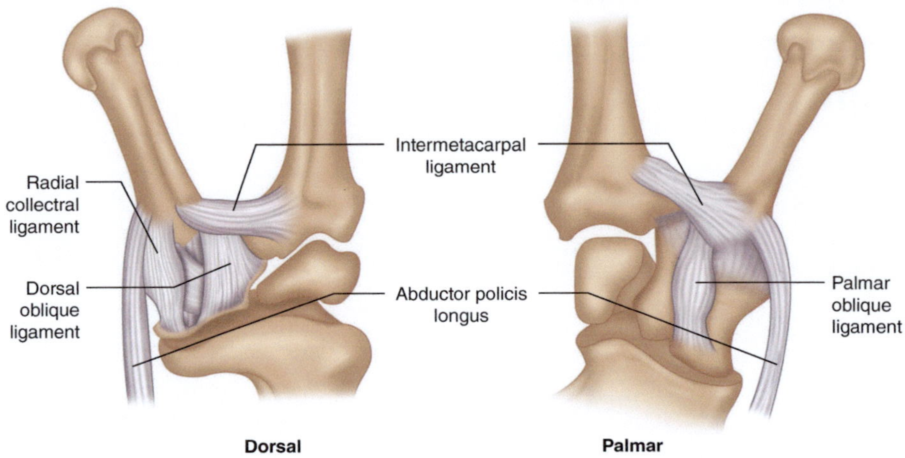

Fig. 1.1 Anatomy of the TMC joint: dorsal and palmar view

The trapezium contains a groove for the FRC as it passes on the way to insert on the volar index metacarpal; the fibrous covering over this groove sometimes ossifies; during trapeziectomy the risk is to damage FRC. The transverse carpal ligament inserts partially on the trapezium trapezoid and the scaphoid; during trapeziectomy it's possible to release the carpal tunnel (Fig. 1.2a–c).

Important elements for TMC joint stability are the beak of the first metacarpal, the recess in the trapezium into which the volar beak inserts and the dorsal ligament complex; this ligament provides the compression to convert the joint from an instable and lax into stable and congruous joint; it cantilevers the volar beak of the thumb metacarpal into the trapezium recess area to permit rotational torque when the thenar intrinsic and thumb flexor muscles actively compress the TM joint into articular congruence during the screw home torque rotation phase of opposition in power grip or power pinch. The intrinsic abductor pollicis brevis muscle abducts the thumb at the TM joint. The opponens pollicis then rotates the thumb so that the flexor brevis, adductor pollicis and flexor pollicis longus can further compress the TM joint. A previously lax, subluxable, incongruous TM joint thus gains articular congruence and rigid stability for power pinch and grasp during the final phase of opposition, the screw home torque rotation. The trapezium recess is the pivot area; the dorsal ligament complex becomes oblique and shortens under tension as the TM joint space is compressed during screw home torque rotation in the last phase of opposition, so that the TM joint converts from gross laxity to powerful stability (Fig. 1.3).

Bettinger et al. at the Mayo Clinic exhaustively identified 16 separate ligaments around the TM joint. The hand surgeon, however, needs to know only principals [4, 5].

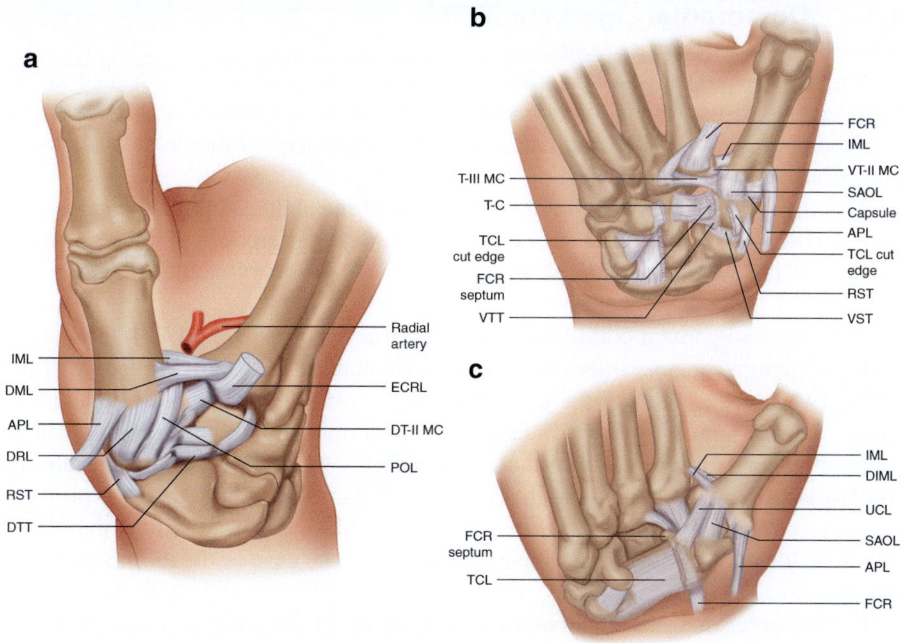

Fig. 1.2 (**a–c**) Dorsal ligaments of TCM joint, deep volar ligaments and superficial volar ligaments

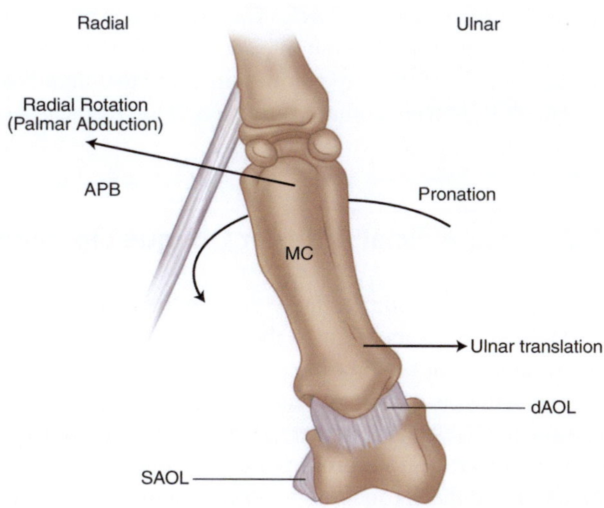

Fig. 1.3 The beak ligament prevents excessive ulnar subluxation of the base of first mtc bone in continued abduction loading. In wide palmar abduction, other TMC ligaments are lax; further motion at the TMC joint is possible in the form of pronation about the axis of the dAOL with continued abduction and flexion

1.1 Dorsoradial Ligament (DRL)

This is the thickest, largest and strongest ligament of the thumb, it attached to the trapezium, it arises from the dorsoradial tubercle of the trapezium, and its insertion is at the dorsal base of the first metacarpal. It's composed of the dorsal radial and posterior oblique subligaments.

This ligament lies adjacent to the dorsal side of the abductor pollicis longus.

The DRL resists the dorsal or dorsoradial subluxating forces in all joint position, except for TM joint extension [4–8], and it acts as a primary stabilizer of the TM joint.

If the dorsal ligament complex is cut or torn (as occurs in a pure TM dislocation without fracture or sometimes in a Bennett's fracture dislocation), gross instability of the TM joint results, and the joint dislocates; even if the volar beak ligament is intact, the TM joint will still dislocate; the dorsal ligament complex contains both longitudinal and oblique portions that create stability when the metacarpal rotates in the TM joint. Strauch concluded that the dorsal ligament complex was the primary restraint to dorsal dislocation and that the volar beak ligament, in effect, permitted dorsal dislocation by stripping subperiosteally from the base of the thumb metacarpal in a pure TM dislocation [6].

Furthermore, the great innervation of this ligament demonstrates that DRL has an important proprioceptive active role in stabilizing the TM joint [6, 8–11], and an increased organization of collagen fibres gives it also a structural advantage [11].

1.2 Posterior Oblique Ligament (POL)

The POL has a large attachment to the dorsal and ulnar edge of the trapezium, immediately ulnar to the DRL. The insertion is at the dorsal-ulnar aspect of the first metacarpal, proximal to the intermetacarpal ligament. Its fibres run obliquely from the dorsal side of the trapezium to insert to the ulnar base of the first metacarpal.

The POL prevents ulnar translation of the metacarpal base during opposition and abduction.

1.3 Superficial Anterior Oblique Ligament (sAOL)

This ligament lies immediately deep to the thenar musculature.

The sAOL has its origin at the volar tubercle of the trapezium, and it inserts over the volar edge of the first metacarpal base.

The sAOL is a capsular ligament and thins down at its edges to blend into the capsule itself, especially at its radial margin. The course of the fibres runs in a slightly oblique direction from proximoradial to distal ulnar. This ligament limits volar subluxation in either pronation, neutral or supination. Short of maximal extension, this ligament appeared lax and redundant regardless of the amount of articular thinning or frank eburnation on either side of the joint. This may represent normal and appropriate laxity to allow for the pronation component of thumb opposition to occur.

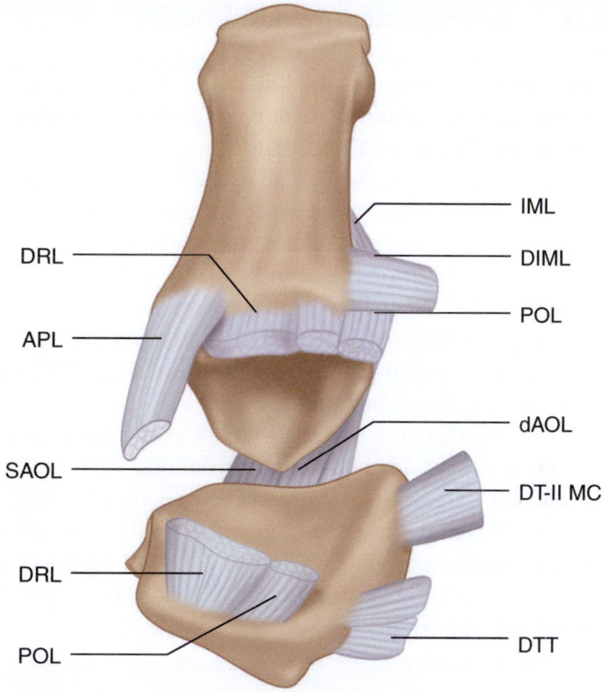

Fig. 1.4 The joint view is from dorsal; it's possible to view the beak ligament (dAOL)

1.4 Deep Anterior Oblique Ligament (dAOL)

This ligament lies deep to the sAOL and it is an intra-articular ligament. Its origin lies proximally on the ulno-volar edge of the base of the trapezium. Distally the dAOL inserts to the articular ulno-volar edge of the styloid process (volar beak) of the thumb metacarpal. For this reason it is also called beak ligament [12] (Fig. 1.4).

Its intra-articular position makes also possible to see it from the intracapsular approach.

It resists to ulnar subluxating forces during abduction and also prevents volar subluxation of the base of the fist metacarpal [13, 14].

Together with the DRL, the dAOL is a primary stabilizer of the TM joint.

During the phase of opposition in power pinch or in power grasp, this ligament is lax; it's tensioned when the thumb is placed in the hitch-hiker position.

The dAOL (beak ligament) shares the responsibility with the sAOL of stabilizing volar metacarpal subluxation.

1.5 Ulnar Collateral Ligament (UCL)

The UCL origins proximal from the distal margin of the transverse carpal ligament and the trapezial ridge, and it inserts on the ulno-volar tubercle of the first metacarpal, adjacent to the intermetacarpal ligaments and superficial and ulnar to the sAOL.

1.6 Intermetacarpal Ligaments

There are two intermetacarpal ligaments that have a role in stabilizing the TM joint: the dorsal first-second metacarpal ligament (D1-2IM) and the volar first-second metacarpal ligament (V1-2IML).

The D1-2IML attached radial to the dorsal-ulnar edge of the first metacarpal base and ulnar at the dorsoradial aspect of the second metacarpal, immediately adjacent to the extensor carpi radialis longus attachment.

The dorsal first intermetacarpal artery (a branch of the radial artery) runs superficial to the D1-2IML.

The attachment of V1-2IML radially lies on the radio-volar base of the first metacarpal, adjacent to the dorsal attachment of the UCL, and ulnarly on the radio-volar base of the second metacarpal.

These two ligaments resist to displacing forces on the base of the first metacarpal, preventing radial and volar translation.

The DTT ligament is capsular; it runs in a transverse direction. The DTT ligament stabilizes the trapezium against cantilever bending forces by resisting trapezial extension and radial deviation. The DTT ligament secures the trapezium to the trapezoid, which is keyed into the second metacarpal. In addition, it resists pronation of the trapezium.

1.7 The Flexor Carpi Radialis and the Flexor Carpi Radialis Groove

The FCR tendon passes volar to the scapho-trapezium-trapezoid joint, and it heads on to insert on the index metacarpal base. The FCR is a convenient and expendable tendon for tenodesis reconstruction of unstable TMC joint after trapeziectomy.

The importance of ligaments is still controversial in literature; Pellegrini considered the beak ligament a key ligament in TMC joint stability; Edmunds in 2011 stressed the importance of the dorsal complex; in fact in author's opinion, it is the most important to guaranty stability during opposition of the thumb. Edmund concluded that the volar beak ligament is taut only when the thumb is in the hitch-hiker position. If the volar beak ligament is severed but the dorsal ligament complex is left intact, the screw home torque rotation mechanism still stabilizes the TM joint by tensioning the dorsal ligament complex to drive the volar beak into its recess in the trapezium for rigid stability. During power pinch and grasp, the abductor pollicis brevis, opponens pollicis, adductor pollicis and flexor pollicis longus drive the volar beak of the thumb metacarpal into the volar recess of the trapezium in the last phase of opposition, so that it can rotate during screw home torque rotation. If the dorsal ligament complex remains intact, even if the volar beak ligament is completely severed, screw home torque rotation stability of the TM joint remains during opposition for power grip and power pinch.

The TM joint presents a challenge to clinicians because of its inherent predisposition for OA disease; one of the potential contributors to progressive OA could be a failure of proprioception and neuromuscular control of the joint.

Ligaments that are continuously subjected to high compressive loads have been shown to have a predominance of Pacinian corpuscles, which are rapidly adapting receptors activated primarily by joint compression [15, 16]; the Ruffini ending is a slowly adapting and constantly active receptor sensitive to axial stress and tensile strains [17, 18]. It has been found to be the dominant mechanoreceptor ending in the wrist ligaments and was similarly the predominant type found in the dorsal TM ligaments. Studies on the kinematic and kinetic functions of the TM joint have shown that motion occurs mostly from translation of the first metacarpal on the trapezium, with large compressive forces transferred across the joint during pinch and grip loading [19]. These compressive forces are located primarily in the volar-ulnar region of the trapezium during functional tasks [20] and result in a tendency for dorsoradial subluxation of the first metacarpal on the trapezium. Considering this, maintained integrity of the dorsal ligament complex is important in maintaining joint congruity, and dorsoradial subluxation has also been implied as a risk factor in the development of TM OA [8].

The presence of Ruffini endings signaling axial strains and tensile forces in the dorsal ligament complex, with predominance in the mobile metacarpal portion of the ligaments, appears logical because this corresponds with the restraining function of the dorsal ligament complex. That the dorsal ligaments are significantly more densely innervated than the volar ligaments infers their importance as primary stabilizers of the TM joint, both from a sensory and a biomechanical perspective. The overall predominance of sensory nerve endings in the dorsal ligaments may also explain the dorsal joint pain frequently encountered in patients with basal thumb OA. A recently proposed explanation for why TM OA is predominantly a female disease has been hormonal influences and the presence of relaxin receptors in the thumb ligaments, which contribute to increased ligament laxity and which, in turn, may predispose to progression of OA [21].

References

1. Pellegrini VD Jr (2005) The ABJS 2005 Nicolas Andry Award: osteoarthritis and injury at the base of the human thumb: survival of the fittest? Clin Orthop Relat Res 438:266–276
2. Acheson RM, Chan YK, Clemett AR (1970) New Haven surgery of joint diseases. XII. Distribution and symptoms of osteoarthrosis in the hands with references to handedness. Ann Rheum Dis 29:275–286
3. Pieron AP (1973) The mechanism of the first carpometacarpal joint: an anatomical and mechanical analysis. Acta Orthop Scand Suppl 148:1–104
4. Bettinger PC, Berger RA (2001) Functional ligamentous anatomy of the trapezium and trapeziometacarpal joint (gross and arthroscopic). Hand Clin 17:151–168
5. Bettinger PC, Linscheid RL, Berger RA, Cooney WP III, An KN (1999) An anatomic study of the stabilizing ligaments of the trapezium and trapeziometacarpal joint. J Hand Surg Am 24:786–798

6. Strauch RJ, Behrman MJ, Rosenwasser MP (1994) Acute dislocation of the carpometacarpal joint of the thumb: an anatomic and cadaver study. J Hand Surg Am 19:93–98
7. Najima H, Oberlin C, Alnot JY, Cadot B (1997) Anatomical and biomechanical of the pathogenesis of trapeziometacarpal degenerative arthritis. J Hand Surg Br 22:183–188
8. Van Brenk B, Richards RR, Mackay MB, Boynton EL (1998) A biomechanical assessment of ligaments preventing dorsoradial subluxation of the trapeziometacarpal joint. J Hand Surg Am 23:607–611
9. Bosmans B, Verhofstad MH, Gosens T (2008) Traumatic thumb carpometacarpal joint dislocation. J Hand Surg Am 33:438–441
10. Colman M, Mass DP, Draganich LF (2007) Effects of the deep anterior oblique and dorsoradial ligaments on trapeziometacarpal joint stability. J Hand Surg Am 32:310–317
11. Mobargha N, Ludwig C, Ladd AL, Hagert E (2014) Ultrastructure and innervation of thumb carpometacarpal ligaments in surgical patients with osteoarthritis. Clin Orthop Relat Res 472:1146–1154
12. Pellegrini VD Jr (1991) Osteoarthritis of the trapeziometacarpal joint: the pathophysiology of articular cartilage degeneration. I Anatomy and pathology of the aging joint. J Hand Surg Am 16:967–974
13. Imaeda T, An K, Cooney W et al (1993) Anatomy of trapeziometacarpal ligaments. J Hand Surg Am 18:226–231
14. Niebur G, Imaeda T, An K-N (1993) Ligament activity of the first carpometacarpal joint. In: Langrana N, Friedman M, Good E (eds) Bioengineering conference. American Society of Mechanical Engineers, Colorado, pp 580–583
15. Johansson H, Sjolander P, Sojka P (1991) A sensory role for the cruciate ligaments. Clin Orthop 268:161–178
16. Moraes MR, Cavalcante ML, Leite JA, Ferreira FV, Castro AJ, Santana MG (2008) Histomorphometric evaluation of mechanoreceptors and free nerve endings in human lateral ankle ligaments. Foot Ankle Int 29:87–90
17. Grigg P (2001) Properties of sensory neurons innervating synovial joints. Cells Tissues Organs 169:218–225
18. Grigg P, Hoffman AH (1996) Stretch-sensitive afferent neurons in cat knee joint capsule: sensitivity to axial and compression stresses and strains. J Neurophysiol 75:1871–1877
19. Cooney WP III, Chao EY (1977) Biomechanical analysis of static forces in the thumb during hand function. J Bone Joint Surg Am 59:27–36
20. Ateshian GA, Ark JW, Rosenwasser MP, Pawluk RJ, Soslowsky LJ, Mow VC (1995) Contact areas in the thumb carpometacarpal joint. J Orthop Res 13:450–458
21. Hagert E, Lee J, Ladd AL (2012) Innervation pattern in trapeziometacarpal joints ligaments. J Hand Surg Am 37:706–714

2 Physical and Radiological Evaluation

2.1 Physical Evaluation

The trapeziometacarpal (TM) joint represents one of the most common sites of osteoarthritis, mostly in the postmenopausal female population [1].

Patients suffering from TM osteoarthritis develop a radial-sided wrist and hand pain. This pain usually is described as a constant ache that increases during normal daily living activities such as gripping, twisting and pinching.

Furthermore patients could complain about a change of appearance of the thumb with a progressive deformity characterized by metacarpal adduction and hyperextension of the metacarpophalangeal joint, as it happens above all in the advanced stages.

Since several causes different from TM osteoarthritis could lead to a radial-sided pain (Table 2.1), a complete and careful clinical evaluation must be performed in order to achieve the correct diagnosis and to assess a correct treatment.

At the inspection, while in the advanced stages, there is the typical deformation above-mentioned, in the early stages the joint appears normal and also the range of motion.

In advanced stages a prominence at the base of the thumb could be present, and it may be due to a synovitis or to a subluxation of the base of the metacarpal to the trapezium or to an osteophyte resulting from the degenerative process.

Usually patients localize the pain palmarly at the base of the thenar eminence of the thumb, and it could be elicited by a manual pressure of this point.

In the early stages, the typical instability of the TM joint could be detected by stabilizing the trapezium and translating the metacarpal in dorso-volar and in a radio-ulnar way, and this manoeuvre results in an abnormal movement of this joint.

Furthermore, applying an axial force during an ulno-radial translation of the TM joint (grind test) could be considered as a provocative manoeuvre since it could elicit pain or discomfort since this manoeuvre increases shear stress at the joint.

S. Odella, *Trapeziometacarpal Joint Osteoarthritis*,
https://doi.org/10.1007/978-3-319-44336-2_2

Table 2.1 Main possible differential diagnosis in radial-sided wrist pain

Diagnosis	Clinical examination
De Quervain's tenosynovitis	Pain over the first extensor compartment; Finkelstein test positive
Scaphoid injuries	Pain over the anatomical snuffbox that increases during movement of flexion and extension of the wrist
Scapho-trapezium-trapezoidal osteoarthritis	Pain distal to the scaphoid

An objective and complete evaluation of the thumb must be performed comparing its movement and key pinch force with the contralateral side. In fact, the range of motion usually is diminished; correlating with the degree of degeneration of the joint and key pinch force is not only diminished but also elicits pain.

In very advanced stage of the disease, the physical features change. In fact it is no more possible to assess the laxity of the TM joint because the degenerative process leads to the formation of osteophytes making it stiff. At the inspection, also the normal shape of the thumb changes since the base of the first metacarpal is placed in dorsal subluxation, and it is fixed in adduction. This fact leads to a loss of range of motion in abduction and adduction and to a compensatory metacarpal-phalangeal hyperextension and a flexion of the interphalangeal joint (due to the effect of the flexor pollicis longus) that produces a Z-shaped deformity.

2.2 Radiographic Evaluation

The radiographic evaluation of the TM joint is usually performed by standard anteroposterior (AP), lateral and oblique X-rays. Dynamic stress view is not usually routinely performed, but it may be used to confirm the diagnosis.

The AP view, also called Robert's view [2], must be obtained by fully pronating the forearm and the shoulder internally rotated and placing the dorsal surface of the thumb next to the X-ray plate (Fig. 2.1).

This way it is possible to clearly evaluate all the trapezial articular facets and also the trapeziometacarpal osteophytes.

The lateral view, also called Gedda's or Bett's view [3], is obtained with the forearm flat on the table, the hand pronated of 20° with the thumb flat on the X-ray plate and the tube angled 10° from the vertical in distal-to-proximal projection. It gives a full view of the trapezium and of the trapeziometacarpal space (Fig. 2.2).

The dynamic stress view is an AP view performed with the radial side of the thumb tips pressing together. It is performed only in case of clinically painful TM joint without degenerative signs at the standard views.

The aim of the dynamic view is to demonstrate a hypermobility or an instability at the TM joint through the demonstration of the dorsoradial subluxation of the metacarpal base.

Several classifications for the TM osteoarthritis were presented, but the most used is Eaton-Littler classification, which is a descriptive system of classification.

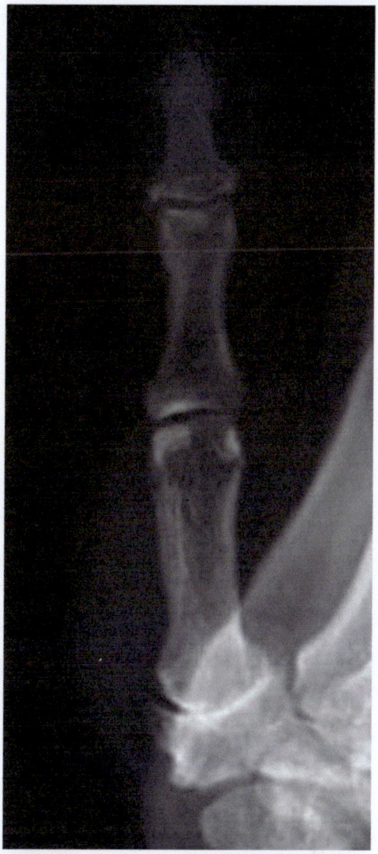

Fig. 2.1 The AP view, also called Robert's view, obtained by fully pronating the forearm and the shoulder internally rotated and placing the dorsal surface of the thumb next to the X-ray plate

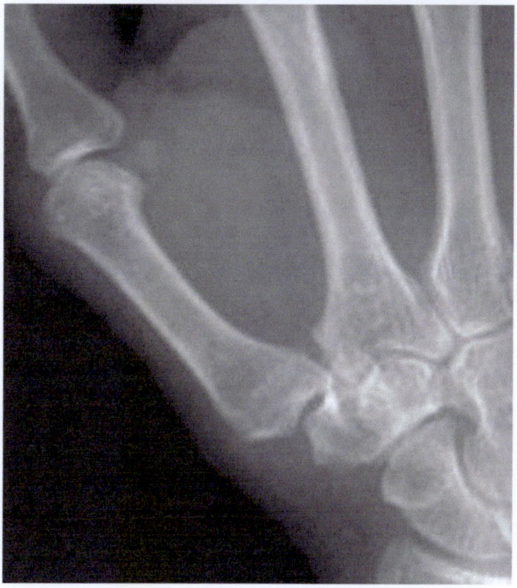

Fig. 2.2 The lateral view, also called Gedda's or Bett's view, gives a full view of the trapezium and of the trapeziometacarpal space

In 1973, Eaton and Littler [4] first described a classification system based on the evaluation of the lateral view, dividing all cases in four stages:

- Stage I: normal or slightly widened TM joint, TM subluxation up to one-third of the articular surface, normal articular contours (Fig. 2.3)
- Stage II: decreased TM joint space, TM subluxation up to one-third of the articular surface, osteophyte or loose bodies <2 mm (Fig. 2.4)

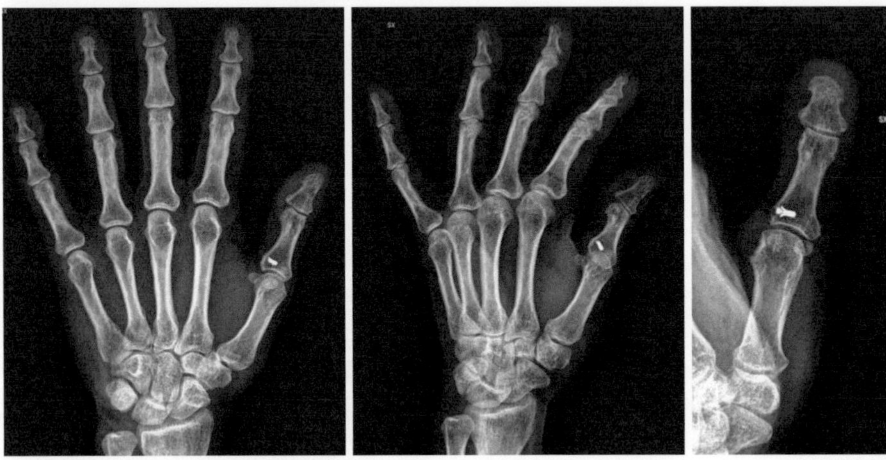

Fig. 2.3 Stage I: normal or slightly widened TM joint, TM subluxation up to one-third of the articular surface, normal articular contours

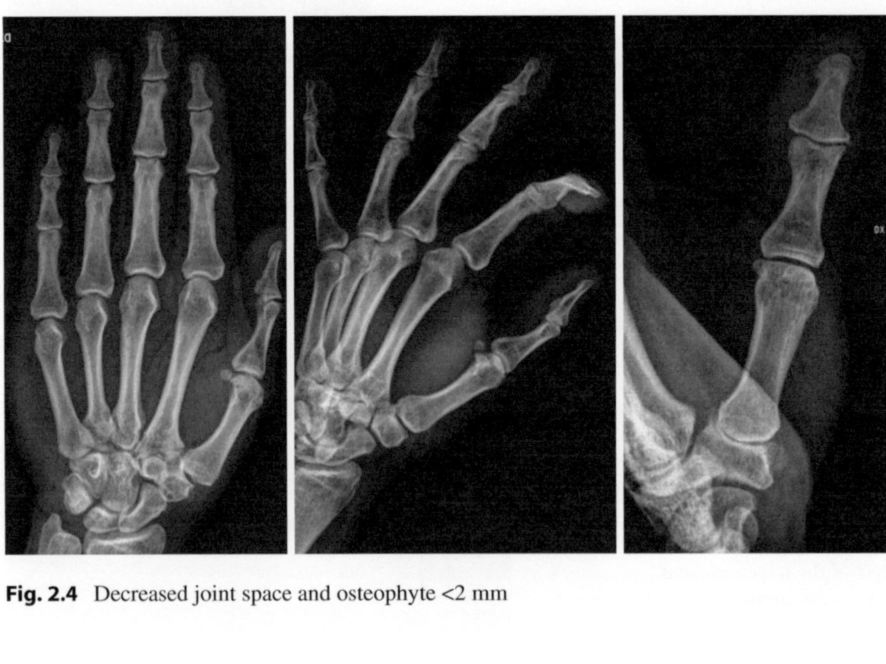

Fig. 2.4 Decreased joint space and osteophyte <2 mm

- Stage III: decreased TM joint space, TM subluxation more than one-third of the articular surface, osteophytes or loose bodies >2 mm, presence of subchondral cysts or sclerosis (Fig. 2.5)
- Stage IV: involvement of the scaphotrapezial joint or, less commonly, of the trapeziotrapezoid joint or of the trapeziometacarpal joint of the second finger (Fig. 2.6)

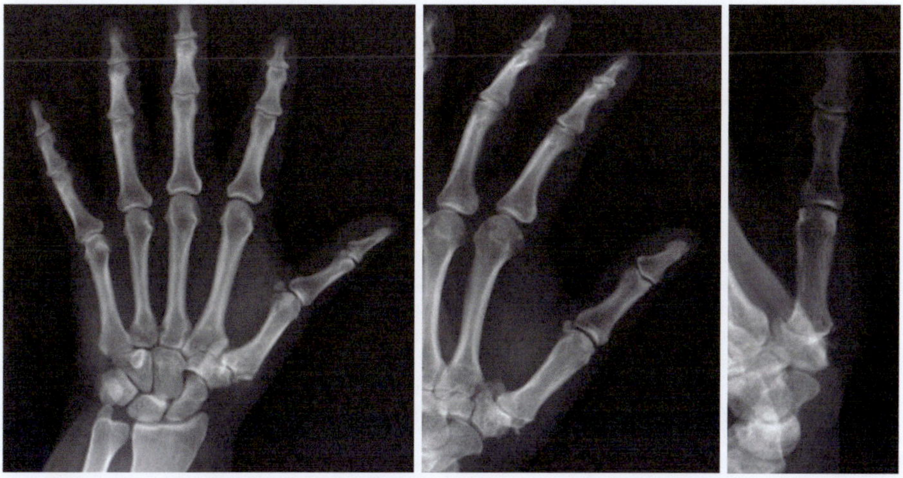

Fig. 2.5 Stage III: subluxation > than 1/3 of the articular surface, subchondral sclerosis, osteophyte >2 mm

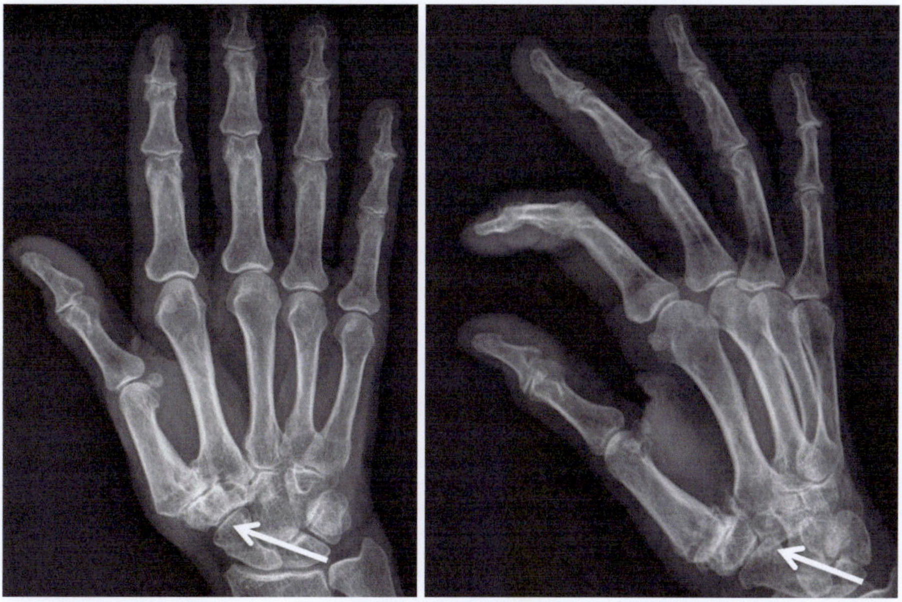

Fig. 2.6 IV stage: involvement of the scaphotrapezial joint

This staging system is widely used nowadays, and it is helpful in preoperative planning, but, however, the divisions in the four stages are not always simple, and there is a clinical overlap between the groups.

Furthermore the radiographic stage is not always correlated to clinical symptoms, and as a proof, about 28% of women who have radiographical features of TM osteoarthritis complain about them [5].

Other methods of radiological evaluation, such as CT and MRI, are rarely used, since they do not give further information about TM osteoarthritis and for preoperative planning.

References

1. Pellegrini VD (2005) The ABJS 2005 Nicolas Andry Award: osteoarthritis and injury at the base of the thumb: survival of the fittest? Clin Orthop Relat Res 438:266–276
2. Robert P (1936) Bullettins et memoires de la Societe de Radiologie Medicale de. France 24:687
3. Billing L, Gedda K (1952) Roentgen examination of Bennett's fracture. Acta Radiol 38:471–476
4. Eaton RG, Littler JW (1973) Ligament reconstruction for the painful thumb carpometacarpal joint. J Bone Joint Surg Am. 55:1655–1666
5. Armstrong AL, Hunter JB, Davis TR (1994) The prevalence of degenerative arthritis of the base of the thumb in post-menopausal women. J Hand Surg Br. 19(3):340–341

Etiopathology

3

Despite the clinical and the various possibilities of treatment of osteoarthritis of the trapeziometacarpal joint that are largely described in literature, the cause of the onset of this pathology is still not completely clear with a lack of paper dedicated to the etiopathology.

The TM osteoarthritis is a pathology caused by several factors.

Genetic, overuse, joint instability, ligamentous laxity, hypermobility of the thumb, anatomical variation of trapeziometacarpal joint (Fig. 3.1) and also particular fractures (e.g. Bennett's fracture, Fig. 3.2) are considered as the main causes of TM osteoarthritis.

The prevalence of TM arthritis, 1/3 of female and 1/8 of male population [1], suggests that there is also a hormonal influence on the pathologic process of cartilage and collagenous tissues.

Compressive loads and shear forces act on the saddle and incongruent articular surface of the TM joint that has no bony constraint, but it is stabilized only by several ligaments.

Biomechanical studies demonstrated that during pinch, the forces transmitted through the thumb at the TM joint are amplified 13 times if compared to the tip of the thumb [2, 3].

The intrinsic instability of the TM joint and the high displacing forces applied to this level highlight the importance of ligament integrity to prevent TM osteoarthritis. The stability is dependent on dynamic and static factors: static stability is provided by joint capsule and ligaments; Bettinger described 16 ligaments around the joint, the most important are the anterior oblique ligament (AOL), the intermetacarpal ligament (IML) and the dorsoradial ligament (DRL); the dynamic stability is provided by tendons that cross the joint (Fig. 3.3).

Several authors tried to understand the etiopathology of TM arthritis considering the biomechanics and the (ligamentous) stabilizer of this joint.

S. Odella, *Trapeziometacarpal Joint Osteoarthritis*,
https://doi.org/10.1007/978-3-319-44336-2_3

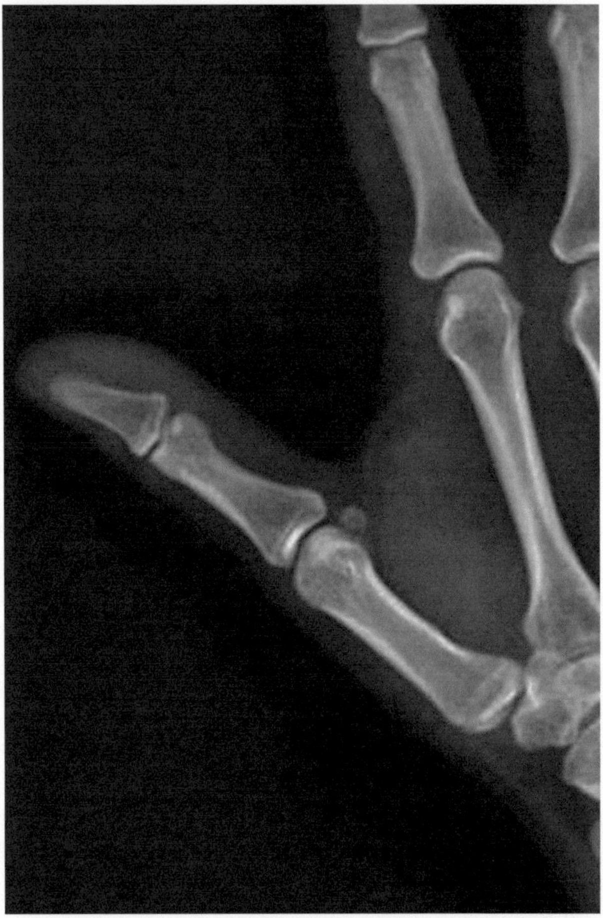

Fig. 3.1 The hypoplasia of the trapezium is a condition that predisposes TMC arthritis

Eaton and Littler stated that compressive loads from the insertion of abductor pollicis longus at the base of the first metacarpal during thumb abduction and extension contribute to TM joint deterioration, since the first part of articular lesion was found to be the dorsoradial facet in most cases [4–6] (Fig. 3.4).

Subsequently, anatomical and pathological studies performed by Pellegrini [7, 8] highlighted as one of the main causes of cartilaginous degeneration the ligamentous laxity; the axial rotation of the first metacarpal depends on a couple force formed by passive ligament tension and active muscle activity and results in an automatic screwing activity; the anterior oblique ligament (AOL, beak ligament) is the pivot for this mechanism; this ligament guides the first metacarpal in pronation, while the thenar muscles work in concert to produce abduction and flexion. This happens

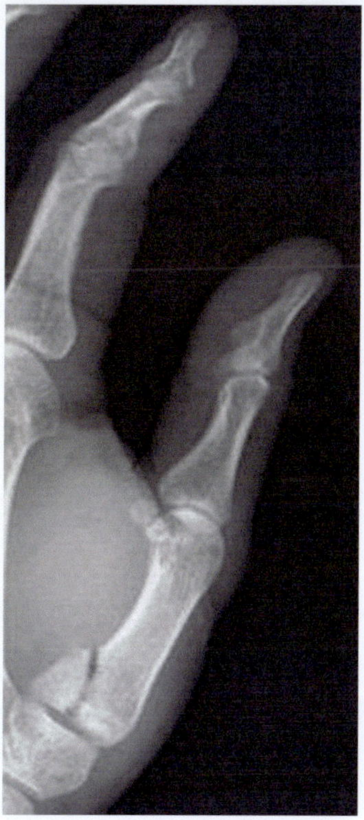

Fig. 3.2 Bennet's fracture involves basal first metacarpal bone; the articular surface could be damage by this kind of trauma, and this condition could predispose the onset of TMC arthritis

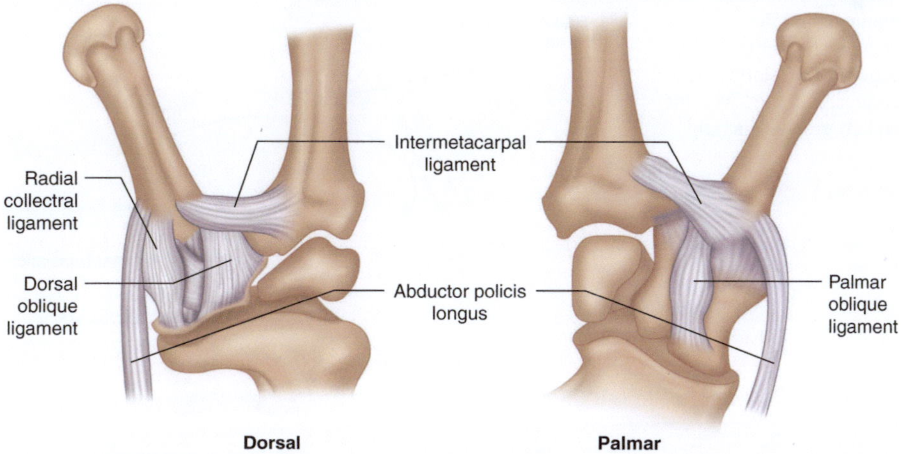

Fig. 3.3 Dorsal and palmar views of TMC joint anatomy: intermetacarpal ligament, palmar oblique ligament and dorsoradial ligament are considered the most important static stabilizers; dynamic stability is provided by tendons that cross the joint

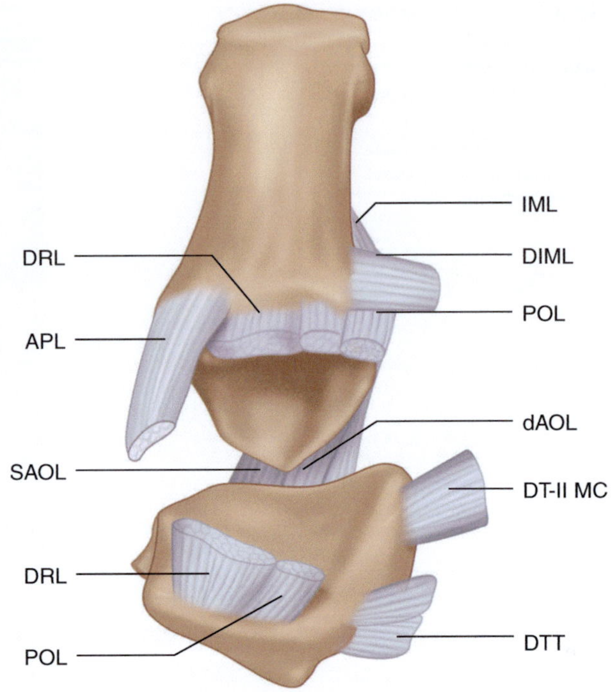

Fig. 3.4 Sixteen ligaments provide the joint stability; APL exerts a traction at the first metacarpal base during thumb abduction and extension that contribute to the joint deterioration; if the APL insertion is more palmar, the dislocating action is greater

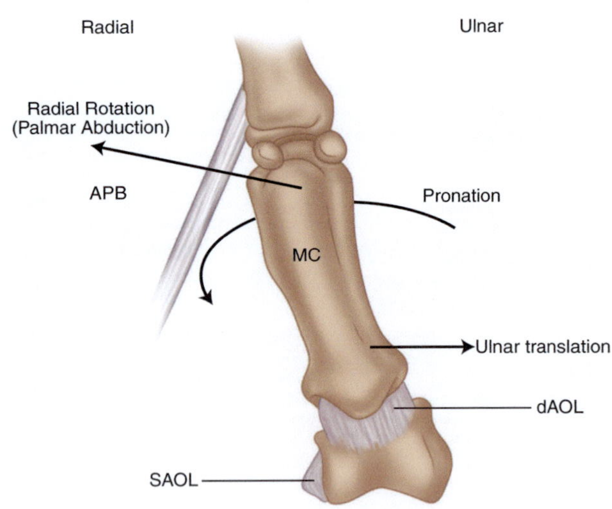

Fig. 3.5 Probably there is a correlation between the integrity of the beak ligament and the degeneration of the joint; degeneration starts at the volar side of the TM joint and progresses dorsally

because the beak ligament is inside the joint, closest to the centre of the joint; its fibres are oriented to limit ulnar translation of the metacarpal during palmar abduction (Fig. 3.5).

Anatomical studies performed on cadaveric human specimens demonstrated that there is a correlation between the integrity of the beak ligament and the degeneration of the articular surface that starts at the volar side of the TM joint and progresses dorsally and usually sparing the dorsal rim of the metacarpal base; the histologic site of beak ligament degeneration in the TMC joint is at the distal or metacarpal attachment, at the fibrocartilaginous insertion zone and within the distal collagen fibres of the ligament. Distal migration and attenuation of the normal zone of insertional fibrocartilage herald progressive articular degeneration.

Once the integrity of the beak ligament is compromised at the metacarpal insertion, complete eburnation of the articular surfaces appears [9].

The presence of a failure of the beak ligament cannot prevent dorsal translation of the metacarpal base during grip and pinch manoeuvres, and it leads to an adduction of the first metacarpal and a compensatory metacarpophalangeal (MCP) hyperextension.

Even though the MCP hyperextension is considered as a compensatory mechanism, caused by loss of motion of the TM joint, forces transmitted during pinch concentrate the load at the palmar side of the TM joint, accelerating the degenerative process [10].

Also articular fractures can lead to TM osteoarthritis with a double mechanism: at first due to the loss of congruence of articular surface and also due to a lesion or a detachment of the beak ligament (as in Bennett's fracture) that leads to destabilization of the thumb base [11].

Bettinger considers the dorsoradial ligament (DRL) an important stabilizer, but the role of this ligament is still controversial [12].

Imaeda [13] stated that the DRL tightens only in extreme supination; it's useful as a checkrein to radial subluxation; it becomes tight in dorsoradial subluxation before any other ligament because it's the shortest ligament spanning the TMC joint.

Another important ligament is the intermetacarpal ligament (IML); it has a common stem at the base of the first ligament and two branches to the second metacarpal bone; Imaeda [13] observed that it's taut in abduction opposition and adduction and it's able to restrain radial subluxation but not dorsal subluxation. Bojsen-Moller hypothesized that the IML is the main stabilizer in the "apoposition": a combination of pronation opposition and flexion used when grasping small things [14].

Besides the above-mentioned causes, there is also a biochemical contribution to the degeneration of hyaline cartilage. Microscopical and biochemical studies [15, 16] evaluated the hyaline cartilage harvested from the volar side of osteoarthritic TM joints.

The extracellular matrix was found to have a preferential loss of glycosaminoglycan with a relative preservation of the collagenous matrix. This preferential degradation, as demonstrated by electron microscopy scanning, reveals a delamination of the superficial layer of the palmar joint surface with a consequent cartilaginous failure.

Harget [17] considers the TMC joint as a synovial organ in which any part of it (cartilage, subchondral bone, synovium, ligaments, nerve, periarticular muscles) can be involved in TMC arthritis. One of the potential causes is the loss of proprioception and neuromuscular control of the joint.

Several authors report a net prevalence of this pathology in Caucasian women from the fifth decade onwards; in a review Pai et al. report a female to male ratio of about 10:1. The sex and gender prevalence suggests a predominant role in post-menopausal hormonal change; considering that thumb OA is a predominantly female disease, a cause of this condition could be a hormonal influence [18, 19]; the presence of relaxin receptors in the thumb ligaments contributes to increase the laxity; ligament laxity has been correlated to reduced joint proprioception. In advance authors found an association with the number of pregnancy and history of past hysterectomy [20].

In early TMC OA, a careful rehabilitation of muscles could be useful to reduce dorsoradial subluxation and instability.

Another factor to be considered is the overuse related to the work activity.

Fontana et al. in 2007 performed a case-control study, and they found an association between a repetitive manual occupation that involves first finger opposition (such as tailor, dressmakers, sewers and domestic helpers) and prevalence of TM joint osteoarthritis [21].

References

1. Armstrong AL, Hunter JB, Davis TRC (1994) The prevalence of degenerative arthritis of the base of the thumb in postmenopausal women. J Hand Surg Br 19:340–341
2. Cooney WP, Chao EY (1977) Biomechanical analysis of static forces in the thumb during hand function. J Bone Joint Surg Am 59:27–36
3. Pellegrini VD, Olcott CW, Hollenberg G (1993) Contact patterns in the trapeziometacarpal joint: the role of the palmar beak ligament. J Hand Surg Am 18:238–244
4. Eaton R, Lane L, Littler JW et al (1984) Ligament reconstruction for the thumb carpometacarpal joint. A long term assessment. J Hand Surg Am 9:692–699
5. Eaton R, Littler JW (1973) Ligament reconstruction for the thumb carpometacarpal joint. J Bone Joint Surg Am 55:1655–1666
6. Eaton R, Littler JW (1969) A study of the basal joint of the thumb. Treatment of its disabilities by fusion. J Bone Joint Surg Am 51:661–668
7. Pellegrini VD Jr (1991) Osteoarthritis of the trapeziometacarpal joint: the pathophysiology of articular cartilage degeneration. I. Anatomy and pathology of the aging joint. J Hand Surg Am 16:967–974
8. Pellegrini VD Jr (1991) Osteoarthritis of the trapeziometacarpal joint: the pathophysiology of articular cartilage degeneration. II. Articular wear patterns in the osteoarthritic joint. J Hand Surg Am 16:975–982
9. Doerschuk SH, Hicks DG, Chinchilli VM, Pellegrini VD Jr (1999) Histopathology of the palmar beak ligament in trapeziometacarpal osteoarthritis. J Hand Surg Am 24(3):496–504
10. Moulton MJ, Parentis MA, Kelly MJ et al (2001) Influence of metacarpophalangeal joint position on basal joint-loading in the thumb. J Bone Joint Surg Am 83:709–716
11. Cullen JP, Parentis MA, Chinchilli VM et al (1997) Simulated Bennett fracture treated with closed reduction and percutaneous pinning: a biomechanical analysis of residual incongruity of the joint. J Bone Joint Surg Am 79:420–423
12. Bettinger P, Linscheid RL, Berger RA, Cooney WP, An KN (1999) An anatomic study of the stabilizing ligaments of the trapezium and trapeziometacarpal joint. J Hand Surg Am 24:786–798
13. Imaeda T, An K-N, Cooney WP III, Linschid R (1993) Anatomy of trapeziometacarpal ligaments. J Hand Surg Am 18:226–231

14. Bojsen-Moller F (1976) Osteoligamentous guidance of the movements of the human thumb. Am J Anat 147:71–80
15. Pellegrini VD Jr, Smith RL, Ku CW (1994) Pathobiology of articular cartilage in trapeziometacarpal osteoarthritis. I. Regional Biochemical analysis. J Hand Surg Am 19:70–78
16. Pellegrini VD Jr, Ku CW, Smith RL (1994) Pathobiology of articular cartilage in trapeziometacarpal osteoarthritis. II. Surface ultrastructure by scanning electron microscopy. J Hand Surg Am 19:79–85
17. Harget E, Lee J, Ladd AL (2012) Innervation patterns of thumb trapeziometacarpal joint ligaments. J Hand Surg Am 37:706–714
18. Wolf JM (2009) The influence of ligamentous laxity and gender: implications for hand surgeons. J Hand Surg Am 34:161–163
19. Pai S, Talwalkar S, Hayton M (2006) Presentation and management of arthritis affecting the trapezio-metacarpal joint. Acta Orthop Belg 72(1):3–10. (Review)
20. Sharma L (2004) The role of proprioceptive deficits, ligamentous laxity, and malalignment in development and progression of knee osteoarthritis. J Reumatol Suppl 70:87–92
21. Fontana L, Neel S, Claise JM, Ughetto S, Catilina P (2007) Osteoarthritis of the thumb carpometacarpal joint in women and occupational risk factors: a case-control study. J Hand Surg Am 32(4):459–465

Non-surgical Treatment

4

Rhizarthrosis is a multifactorial disease caused by different pathological conditions. The alteration of articular cartilage surfaces overtime leads to an instability of the trapeziometacarpal joint (TMJ) leading to pain and functional limitation with progressive loss of strength of the “functional clamp” and the “jack”, up to a significant restriction of the use of the hand [1, 2].

The treatment cannot disregard a correct diagnostic process, that *involves a good clinical examination* and all the possibilities that imaging offers, including diagnostic arthroscopy recently introduced [3].

The most used classification is the Eaton–Littler which divides the disease into four stages [4].

Nowadays surgical treatment is recommended in the fourth stage and sometimes in the third.

It certainly gives better results than in the past, but some doubts are still left on the choice of intervention and we should consider in any case the incidence of surgical of complications [5].

In the first two stages of Eaton’s classification, conservative treatment is more advisable. The goals of conservative treatment are:

- Control of pain and inflammation
- A basic treatment for osteoarthritis
- Maintaining a functional range of motion as long as possible
- Delaying surgery countering deformations [6, 7]

Once nonoperative treatment is chosen, due to the extreme variety of the disease associated with its chronicity, the patient has to frame the patient comprehensively by requiring:

- Age, sex and type of functional request:
  - Young people will try in every way to procrastinate surgical treatment, with a multi-year plan of nonoperative treatment.

S. Odella, *Trapeziometacarpal Joint Osteoarthritis*,
https://doi.org/10.1007/978-3-319-44336-2_4

  - A man who performs heavy work may have lower demands than a small woman who uses her hands for delicate work such as sewing. It's also important to assess the needs of the subject in the recreational area: sport, movements, frequency and intensity of sport are also to be considered.
- Pain characteristics:
  - At the onset: morning, evening, after use of the thumb, etc.
  - How it evolves: resolves without medical interventions or physical therapy or medical treatment necessary
  - Intensity and characteristics
- Deformity more or less obvious
- Decreased strength and range of motion [8]

Nonoperative treatment offers a wide variety of possibilities: drug therapy, orthoses, hand therapy, the endoarticular infiltration and finally the combination of all these treatments [2].

4.1 Pharmacological Therapy

The American College of Rheumatology (ADR) in 2012 published guidelines for osteoarthritis of the knee, hip and hand, an update to the guidelines published in 2000 [9].

The nonoperative treatment of osteoarthritis in general and more specifically of TMA makes use of different therapies. The difficulties of physician and different specialists who follow these patients are the choice of strategy, in time, that is necessary for the individual patient [10].

The general practitioner and the specialist have to face endless scenarios of therapies isolated or in combination, often not validated by extensive studies. The ADR report is the result of bibliographical studies and evaluations of different specialists. In particular, for the hand, they have drawn to the recommendations of EULAR for the treatment of osteoarthritis [11–13].

The ARD for osteoarthritis of the hand, as for the other localizations, gives recommendations "strong" or "under investigation". These recommendations do not want to be rules but a guide based on clinical evidence and an advice by medical experts in this field, with which to be compared.

- *Strong recommendation to use*: a recommendation is strong if scientific evidences are of high quality and if the probability of a desirable effect (benefit) exceeds that of an adverse effect.
- *Weak or subject to recommendation:* if the recommendation is weak, the patient will tend not to choose it; the doctor will examine, based on local and general conditions, whether to recommend or not the patient performing the treatment.
- *Strong recommendation not to use*: it would not be prescribing.

These recommendations will be used by the attending physician to set a course of treatment with the patient if he will give his consensus after extensive and detailed interview.

4.1.1 Drug Treatment in the Early Stages

The experts recommend "conditional" that patients with osteoarthritis of the hand have been handled:

- With NSAIDs topically.
- With oral NSAIDs including selective COX-2 inhibitors.
- Capsaicin topically.
- Tramadol.
- Recommended "conditional" to treat these patients with analgesics.
- Opiates or with intra-articular therapies.
- For patients with joint involvement trapeziometacarpal and requiring an intra-articular injection, experts recommend "conditional" not to use corticosteroids or hyaluronic acid intra-articularly; it also does not express a preference between these two treatments in the case in which the physician chooses injection as therapy.
- In case of patients over 75 years old, it's recommended the use of NSAIDs topically.

Note1. Experts do not give "strong" recommendations for treatment of pharmacological osteoarthritis of the hand.

Note 2. For patients with erosive interphalangeal osteoarthritis and/or inflammatory osteoarthritis, experts recommend "conditional" not to use methotrexate or sulphasalazine orally and have chosen not to express themselves for or against the use of hydroxychloroquine [9].

In acute phases, the thumb root looks swollen and red, with important functional limitation and, above all, highly debilitating in the execution of the usual daily actions; the TMC joint is critical to the "pincer" movement. It will also establish the opposition of the thumb to the other fingers.

In our experience at this stage, we treat the patient with NSAIDs, rest and we also recommend the use of orthoses associated or not to endoarticular infiltration and rarely corticosteroids for oral use. It's clear that NSAIDs and the corticosteroids reduce inflammation, synovitis and pain, but it cannot reduce or block the progression of the disease [14].

In the subacute phase, drug treatment is discontinued in favour of the non-drug treatment: orthotics and physical therapy.

In the chronic phase, treatment with drugs for oral use containing precursors of hyaluronic acid like chondroitin sulphate or the glucosamine sulphate may be considered, although the use of these drugs seems controversial [15, 16].

4.1.2 Intra-articular Injection

It is commonly recognized that endoarticular infiltration can reduce pain and inflammation [17].

The endoarticular infiltration of a drug is aimed at increasing the *in loco* pharmacological activity and reducing the general side effects.

The indications are:

- Add on to general drug therapy
- In association with physical therapy
- As painkiller and to reduce synovial flogosys

It is worth noting that the endoarticular anti-inflammatory treatment is not able to slow down the articular aging process.

Similar complications as the ones seen in any other endoarticular treatment are noticed: local/systemic infection, allergic reaction, microcrystalline synovitis and light articular swelling.

Different endoarticular drugs can be used in arthrosis: corticosteroid, NSIAD, hyaluronic acid, orgothein (SOD), some glycosaminoglycan, osmic acid and Yttrio 90.

4.2 TMC Infiltration Technique

The infiltration technique is executed with 1 mL size syringes, high molecular weights hyaluronic Ac with 22 G needle. Before performing the intra-articular injection, a local anesthesia is performed.

To make sure the drug is correctly injected in the articulation, it is possible to perform a fluoroscopic examination [18].

Otherwise it is important to mark the articulation limit.

Marking the palpatory shape of trapezium and I metacarpal adds a visual aid for the introduction of the needle (Fig. 4.1).

It is very important to maintain asepsis during the infiltration using sterile gloves and cutaneous disinfection on needle introduction area (ammonium quaternarium is suggested) (Figs. 4.2, 4.3, and 4.4).

The efficacy of corticosteroid in OA is mainly due to the antiphlogistic effect: both a local inhibition of prostaglandin synthesis and a reduced production of IL-1 and of proteasic-activities enzyme are obtained.

Some systemic activity is left, depending on dosage and solubility of the used product.

Treatment appears to be effective in the short term [20].

The majority of the available research highlights the pain and inflammation reduction observed with endoarticular cortisonic treatment [17].

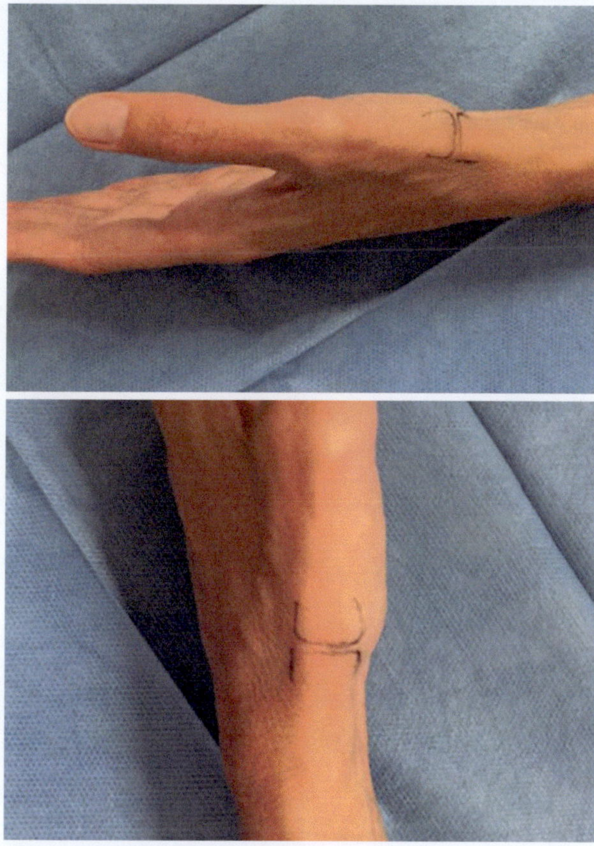

Fig. 4.1 Before endoarticular infiltration, metacarpal and trapezoidal joint extremities must be precisely traced

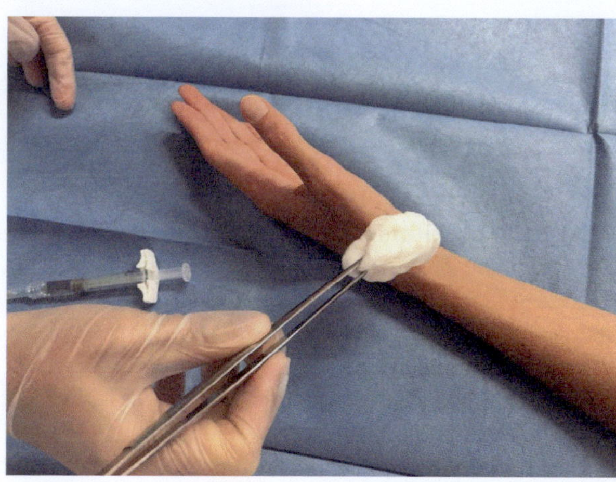

Fig. 4.2 An axial traction is executed on P2 thumb in order to distract the articular extremities

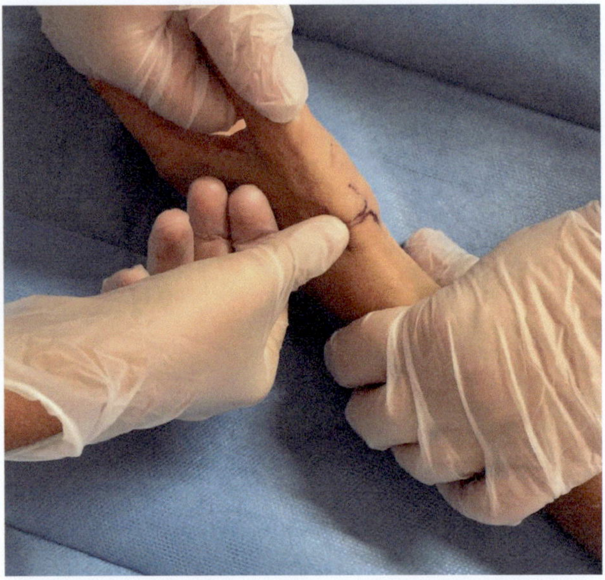

Fig. 4.3 Through palpation of the joint line, the needle is perpendicularly inserted, and when the tactile perception confirms having passed the articular capsule, the drug is injected

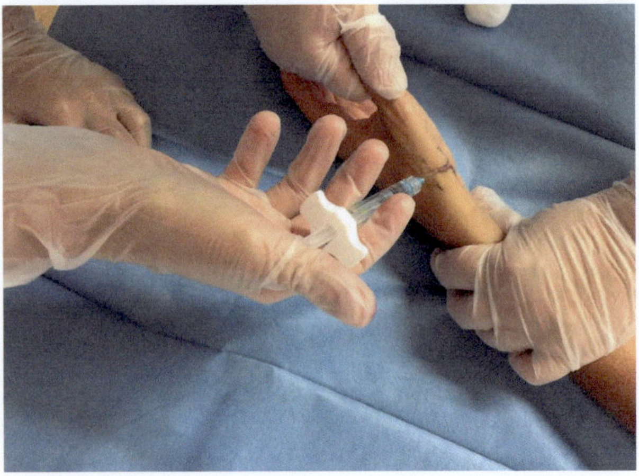

Fig. 4.4 Cortisonic endoarticular infiltration treatment was firstly elaborated by Hollander in 1951 [20]

Different conclusions are drawn: Meenagh reports non-significative difference between corticosteroid and placebo infiltrations through a study vs. placebo.

Contraindications are limited: it's better to avoid steroid injection in presence of articular prosthesis, in case of anticoagulant therapy or hemorrhagic diathesis or non-compensated DM.

Cutaneous atrophy is possible if the drugs are injected in subcutaneous tissue instead of endoarticular space.

The role of corticosteroid articular infiltration on cartilaginous alterations is not clear: destructive arthropathy is rare; articular degeneration is proved not to be related to infiltration through studies on the knee with indirect detection systems [21].

In 1970, Balazs and Denlinger introduced the viscosupplementation or forced lubrication theory, using intra-articular HA to restore the articular viscoelastic condition [22].

The alteration due to arthrosis mainly affects endogenous HA, significantly reducing its concentration.

In consequence, a reduction of HA is obtained, both due to dilution after swelling and to HA degradation in synovial liquid and altered synthesis.

This condition associated with molecular weight and synovial liquid viscosity alterations increases the probability of further damages to the joint surfaces [23].

HA is a polysaccharide chain built from *N*-acetylglucosamine and glucuronic acid, with 4–6 million MW. It fills the intercellular space. It is a highly hydrated polyanion with reticular structure: the distended molecule is 10-μm length. Articular homeostasis highly depends on these molecules [24].

HA represents a basic constituent of the synovial liquid and of the extracellular matrix of the articular cartilage, where it has a very important role. HA synthesis is controlled by three different genes, synthesizing different weight molecules [25].

HA activity depends on its location:

1. At the synovial membrane level, it drives exchanges between hemolymphatic circulation and synovial liquid, it has a protective effect on synoviocytes and nociceptive nervous terminations, and it controls cellular movement with the articular cavity.
2. In the synovial liquid, it controls the solutes distribution, but its main function regards the viscosity control. This property allows the maintenance of a correct lubrication of joint surfaces and dampens and separates them.
3. In the articular cartilage, it performs different functions:
   (a) It is one of the components of the cartilaginous matrix and thus has a shock absorber function.
   (b) It determines the viscosity and elasticity of cartilaginous tissue, since it is an aggregation of proteoglycans, which, being hydrophilic, increase the water content.
   (c) It has an anti-degenerative and anti-inflammatory function because of its inhibition effects on interleukin and metalloproteinase production [MMP] in synovial tissue and on the production of nitrous oxide [NO] in synovial issue [26–29].

The HA intra-articular infiltration, by increasing the concentration of HA in this region, has three main effects:

- Anti-degenerative action by inhibiting the IL1, NO and MPO production.
- Reconstructive action by stimulating proteoglycans and new HA synthesis.
- Quite immediate analgesic effect, due to its action on nociceptors, blocking the production of algogenic substances. Moreover, it has a long-term analgesic effect due to a better articular homeostasis. The improvement of the articular condition allows maintaining benefits on the long term, even in case of exogenous HA persistence for a few hours to a maximum of several days [30, 31].

Many different HA preparations are available on the market: apart from different composition modalities, these present with different molecular weights. Since viscoelastic properties are related to the molecular weight, treatment can be modulated by changing the formulation. Higher MW generally have mechanical effects, while medium MW have better biologic function [32–36].

In rhizarthrosis, inflammation changes joint homeostasis by increasing HA degradation. Thus, also in this articulation, HA infiltrations help improving articular homeostasis. Treatment is performed by the introduction of HA hydrogel, MW 1.2 × 10 million Da, in pre-filled syringe.

The number and frequency of treatment vary depending on the author. Generally, 3–6 infiltrations are suggested once a week, even though Roux et al. have studied three patient groups with different frequency: in the first group, once a week administration was performed; in the second group, twice a week administration was performed; and in the third group, administration was done three times a week. After 3 months, all the patients showed an improvement in pain relief [37].

Many studies compared the results of HA infiltrative treatment versus corticosteroid infiltration.

The choice of the drug type depends on its painkiller effect and the effectiveness in maintaining the pain reduction.

Corticosteroid infiltrations surely have a faster effect as painkillers, while HA has a longer action due to multiple effects in the articular location (analgesic effect and chondroprotective activity, viscosupplementation mechanical activity, antiphlogistic effect) [35–39].

In conclusion, we believe that an infiltrative treatment has both pain and inflammation reduction action. It is advisable to perform it in early stages (Eaton phase 1/2). It is safe and can be repeated. Different conclusions are drawn in literature about its efficacy, but we believe that it could be effective by adopting some technical tips and tricks such as using a fluoroscopic guide during the learning curve. The degenerative progression of arthritis progression is clearly not modified by this treatment.

4.2.1 Non-pharmacologic Treatments

There are some expert recommendations subjected to check:

- Every patient affected by osteoarthritis of the hand should be examined by the specialist doctor and not by the general practitioner or by a physiotherapist or occupational physician, about their ability to perform normal daily activities.
- Receive assistive devices if needed.
- Receive advice for joint protection and the use of thermal agents for relief from pain and stiffness.
- Recommended “conditional” that patients with rhizarthrosis should benefit from application of splint [9].

4.3 Orthoses

The indications for the use of a static splint are pain and instability of the joint.

The objectives to be pursued in the use of splints are those of increasing stability, reducing pain, reducing inflammation, increasing the function and reducing mechanical stress.

Initial treatment should include the use of splint that immobilizes wrist and thumb [8, 40, 41].

This treatment is recommended in painful phase, but it can be recommended in every stage of the disease [42].

When the orthosis is able to stabilize the joint, it is obtained a pain relief, but it does not change the joint function as the clamp force, grip and motility.

The pain relief is almost instantaneous by using orthoses that block movement compared to those that allow an articular movement [8, 43].

The orthosis can be differentiated for multiple features:

- Prefabricated or custom-made
- Short or long
- Soft or rigid material
- For daily use

Both custom-made and prefabricated orthoses could reduce pain. A large majority of patients prefer the prefabricated ones, probably for the low cost or for speed in the acquisition [44], although some authors report a more important remission of painful symptomatology with custom-made orthosis [45].

Two-thirds of patients choose shorter orthosis than longer, probably for comfort due to a larger ROM; wherefore, not significant changes in pain reduction are reported [46].

There is a difference of improvement in pain between the splint made with soft material compared to those with rigid material [47].

It's possible using material to be shaped directly on the patient.

It is made with perforated sheets, to allow transpiration, with low thickness (2 mm) and non-allergenic (Fig. 4.5). Once the material becomes stiff, the orthosis are washable and considerably resistant.

This kind of sheets, which it's possible to cut until the wanted size, allows to model the splint directly on the patient's hand.

It's necessary to stabilize both the trapeziometacarpal joint and the metacarpal phalangeal joint of the thumb.

The proximal edge must be 1 cm distally from the radial styloid; fingers and thumb interphalangeal joint must be free. The thumb should be positioned in antepulsion position (40°) and abduction (20°) with the metacarpal phalangeal joint slightly flexed (Fig. 4.6).

Once the sheet has been cut and shaped, you have to use a dryer to make the orthosis rigid.

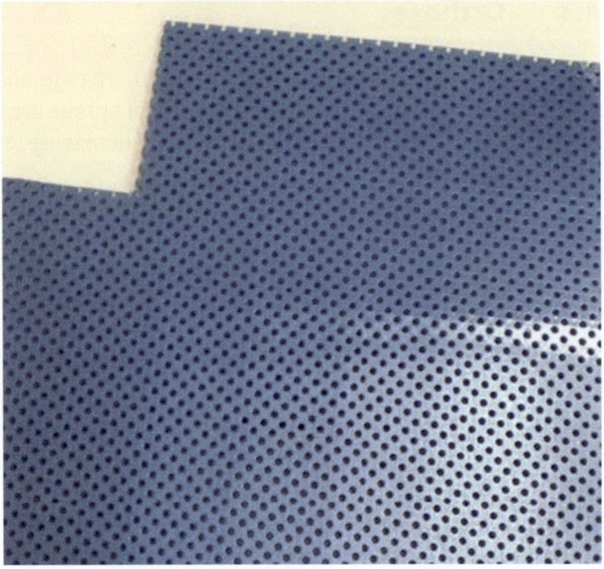

Fig. 4.5 Porous non-allergenic material to build custom-made thumb splint

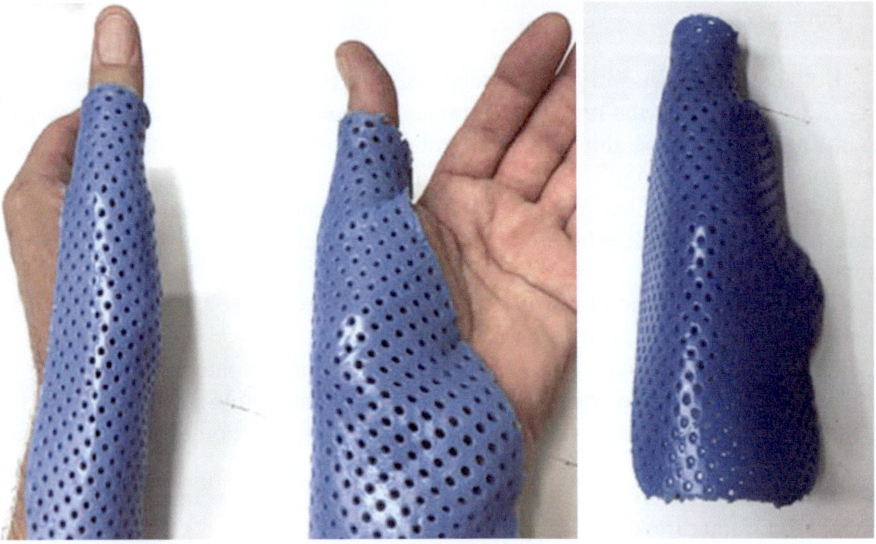

Fig. 4.6 Custom-made thumb splint

The orthosis must be maintained throughout the night and, in the stages of intense pain, even in the daytime, especially to use when it's necessary to run a business who submits the joints affected by stress.

In conclusion, although the use of the orthosis is a recommendation with "Reserve" on the part of the ADR, in our current practice, we use systematically the orthosis in the early stages of osteoarthritis of TM joint, associated with specific gymnastics to prevent joint stiffness and the decrease in strength.

In our practice we use a brace to be shaped on the hand of patient, short, with rigid material, to maintain definitely all night and modulating the use during the day based on the control of pain.

It's a common sense that the use of the orthosis in the early stages of disease makes an important benefit in pain control [8].

4.4 Physical Therapy

4.4.1 Physiotherapy Treatment

Physiotherapy support is essential at every stage of the disease, both for maintaining joint functionality and for reinforcing the musculature.

Physiotherapy support must include:

- Educating the arrangements for strengthening of the thenar muscles
- Allowing the use of the thumb without increasing shear stress
- Massaging that can reduce pain [42]

Physiotherapy treatment is set on two stages:

Education: to teach the patient what can and should do

Domiciliary physical exercises: to strengthen the muscles and maintain the range of motion.

Valdes and Von der Heide [43] suggest these exercise series; each exercise has to performed passively and actively:

Thumb flexion: starting with thumb extended the tip has to be flexed to the base of the small finger as in Fig. 4.7.

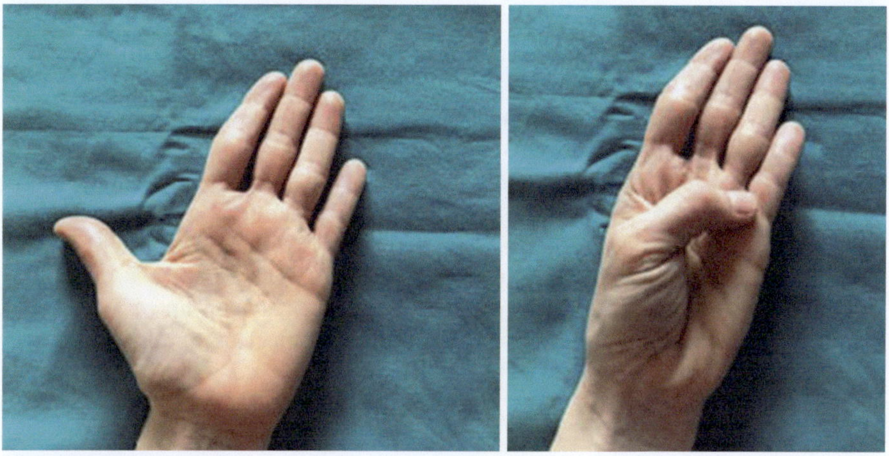

Fig. 4.7 Thumb flexion

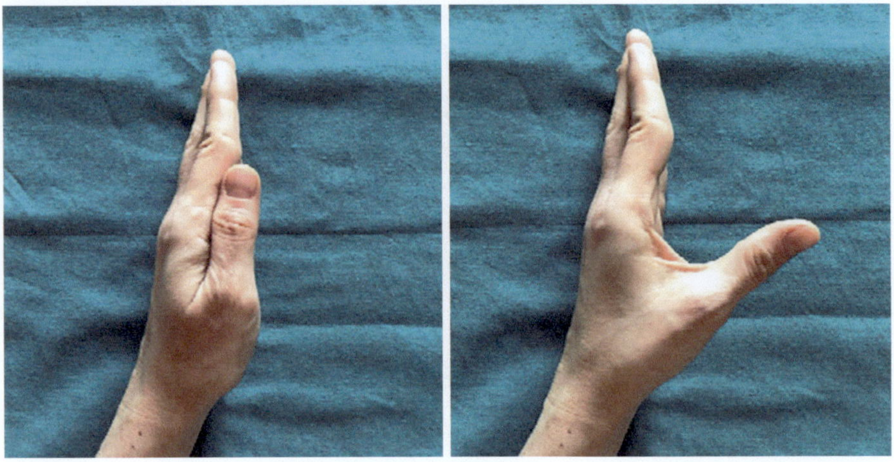

Fig. 4.8 Thumb abduction

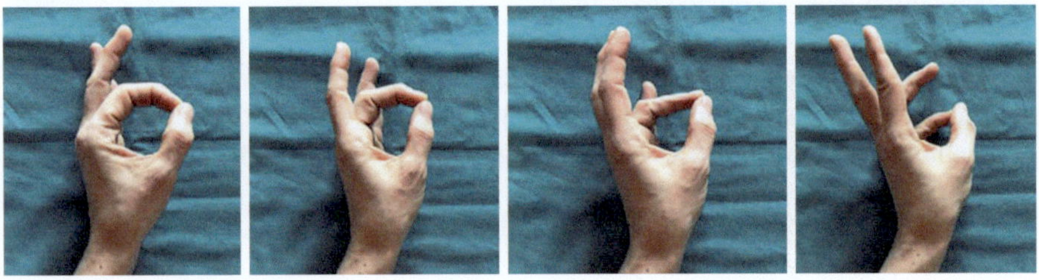

Fig. 4.9 Thumb opposition

Thumb abduction: starting with the thumb against the palm in line with the index finger, spreading it away from the palm as far as possible, in the same line as the index finger (Fig. 4.8).

Thumb opposition: the tip of the thumb touch the tip of each fingertip alternately (Fig. 4.9).

Thumb CMC extension: spreading the thumb far away from the palm avoiding to hyperextend the MP joint (Fig. 4.10).

Thumb IP flexion: bending just the tip of the thumb as in Fig. 4.11.

Exercises should be performed one set for 10–15 repetitions, 2–3 times a week; these exercises must be performed pain free; in case of advanced OA or TMC instability, lateral pinch and key pinch strengthening should be avoided.

Pinch strengthening consists in pinching an object between tip of fingers and thumb; grip strengthening consists in squeezing an object as tightly as possible without inducing pain.

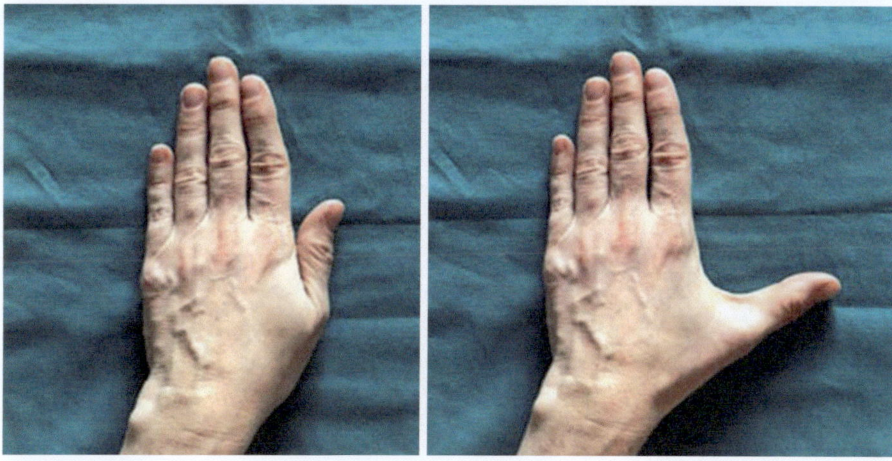

Fig. 4.10 Thumb CMC joint extension

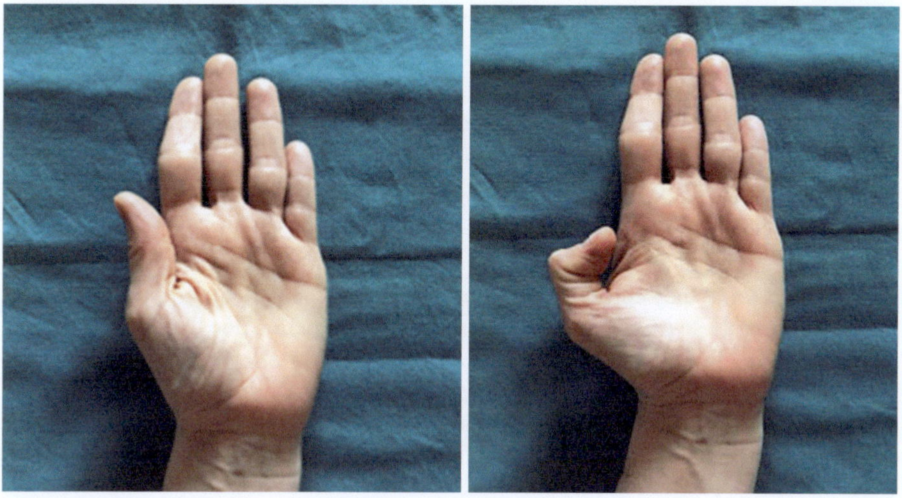

Fig. 4.11 Thumb IP flexion

4.4.2 Education Programme

It is important that the physical therapist evaluates the clinical situation and considers the normal patient activity at his home and at work.

In this way it's possible to teach patients the importance of rest joint at every stage of treatment: removing every movement that can result in inflammation. In this way, in the acute phase we will seek to prevent movement of gripping, rotating and opposition, and teach how to use the other joints and the device to allow an increased protection of the thumb without worsening joint situation.

Table 4.1 Hand exercises [53]

Exercise	Description
Tabletop	The hand and wrist are held in neutral position, subject flexes at the second to fifth metacarpophalangeal (MCP) joints only and then returns to neutral
Small fist	From neutral position, subject flexes at the second to fifth proximal interphalangeal joint and distal interphalangeal joint only and then returns to neutral
Large fist	From neutral position, subject flexes all joint to form a fist and then returns to neutral
Okay signs	From neutral position, subject flexes to form an "O" with the tip of the thumb to the tip of each finger in turn, returning to neutral after each
Finger spread	From neutral position, the hand is placed on flat tabletop and the fingers are spread apart as wide as possible before returning to neutral
Thumb reach	From neutral position, subject reaches across the palm of the hand and touches the tip of the thumb to fifth MCP and then returns to neutral
Gripping	Subject holds the Thera-Band® Hand Exerciser Ball in the palm of the hand and squeezes until the ball is about 50% depressed
Key pinch	Subject holds the Thera-Band® Hand Exerciser Ball between the side of the thumb and side of the index finger and squeezes until the ball is about 50% depressed
Fingertip pinch	Subject holds the Thera-Band® Hand Exerciser Ball between the tip of the thumb and the tip of the index finger and squeezes until the ball is about 50% depressed; this is repeated for digits three to five

When there are no obvious joint deformations, strengthening and flexibility exercises are particularly indicated [48]. We will then try to teach the patient not to subject the ATM joint to excessive loads for a long time. After being properly educated to protect his joint, they certainly have both the benefits and the improvement of pain [49]. Moreover these exercises allow to prevent the adduction due to contracture with reduction of the first intermetacarpal space [50, 51]. The task force of the European anti-rheumatism association advises to perform the recommended exercises daily, even if the lack of in-depth studies does not allow to evaluate the validity of such treatment [52, 53] (Table. 4.1). It is certain that the combination of education program of joint protection associated with specific hand exercises has improved the overall function of the hand and the force of the forceps [54]. It can therefore be concluded that the assistance of expert physiatrists is necessary to maintain the force of the forceps and the range of movement of the thumb as long as possible, by counteracting contractures and joint deformations. The treatment will take place on two different levels: (1) Educational: to teach the movements necessary to avoid further stress to the joint. (2) Practical: daily exercises performed by the patient. There is no certain evidence on these indications but current practice allows us to recommend these therapeutic programs that delay the evolution of the disease.

Physical therapy

- Laser therapy (Laser super pulsed cold or NdYag): the treatment is applied to the trapezius metacarpal joint
- Ultrasound, often used in combination with NSAIDs topically

- Tecar therapy or magnetic therapy
- Kinesio Taping: applications patches mode decongestant to facilitate the reduction of edema in the area

References

1. Gillis J, Calder K, William J (2011) Review of thumb carpometacarpal arthritis classification, treatment and outcomes. Can J Plast Surg 19(4):134–138
2. Spaans AJ, van Minnen LP, Kon M, Schuurman AH, Schreuders AR, Vermeulen GM (2015) Conservative treatment of thumb base osteoarthritis: a systematic review. J Hand Surg [Am] 40:16–21
3. Badia A (2006) Trapeziometacarpal arthroscopy: a classification and treatment algorithm. Hand Clin 22:153–163
4. Eaton RG, Glickel SZ (1987) Trapeziometacarpal osteoarthrits: staging as a rationale for treatment. Hand Clin 3(4):455–471
5. Vermeulen GM, Slijper H, Feitz R, Hovius SER, Moojen TM, Selles RW (2011) Surgical management of primary thumb carpometacarpal osteoarthritis: a systematic review. J Hand Surg [Am] 36(5):157–169
6. Poole JU, Pellegrini VD Jr (2000) Arthritis of the thumb basal joint complex. J Hand Ther 13(2):91–107
7. Berger AJ, Momeni A, Ladd AL (2014) Intra- and interobserver reliability of the Eaton classification for trapeziometacarpal arthritis: a systematic review. Clin Orthop Relat Res 472(4):1155–1159
8. Magnelli L, Oriani M, Delcroix L, Ceruso M. Il trattamento conservativo della rizoartrosi La rizoartrosi. Vol. 1, Casa ed. Mattioli Fidenza;1996. p. 65–74.
9. Hochberg MC, Altman RD, Toupin K, Benkhalti M, Guyatt G, Mcgowan J, Towheed T, Welch V, Wells G, Tugwell P (2012) American College of Rheumatology 2012 recommendations for the use of nonpharmacologic and pharmacologic therapies in osteoarthritis of the hand, hip, and knee. Arthritis Care Res 64(4):465–474
10. Dougados M, Hochberg MC (2011) Management of osteoarthritis. In: Hochberg MC, Silman AJ, Smolen JS, Weinblatt ME, Weisman M (eds) Rheumatology, 5th edn. Mosby/Elsevier, Philadelphia, pp 1793–1799
11. Jordan KM, Arden NK, Doherty M, Bannwarth B, Bijlsma JW, Dieppe P et al (2003) EULAR recommendations 2003: an evidence based approach to the management of knee osteoarthritis: report of a Task Force of the EULAR Standing Committee for International Clinical Studies Including Therapeutic Trials (ESCISIT). Ann Rheum Dis 62:1145–1155
12. Zhang W, Doherty M, Arden N, Bannwarth B, Bijlsma J, Gunther KP et al (2005) EULAR evidence based recommendations for the management of hip osteoarthritis: report of a Task Force of the Standing Committee for International Clinical Studies Including Therapeutic Trials (ESCISIT). Ann Rheum Dis 64:669–681
13. Zhang W, Doherty M, Leeb BF, Alekseeva L, Arden NK, Bijlsma JW et al (2007) EULAR evidence based recommendations for the management of hand osteoarthritis: report of a Task Force of the EULAR Standing Committee for International Clinical Studies Including Therapeutic Trials (ESCISIT). Ann Rheum Dis 66:377–388
14. Brook PM, Day RO (1991) Nonsteroidal anti-inflammatory drugs-differences an similarities. N Engl J Med 342:1716–1725
15. Black C, Clar C, Henderson R, McEachern C, McNamee P, Quayyum Z, Royle P, Thomas S (2099 Nov) The clinical effectiveness of glucosamine and chondroitin supplements in slowing or arresting progression of osteoarthritis of the knee: a systematic review and economic evaluation. Health Technol Assess 13(52):1–148
16. Hochberg M, Chevalier X, Henrotin Y, Hunter DJ, Uebelhart D (2013) Sympton and structure modification in osteoarthritis with pharmaceutical-grade chondroitin sulfate: what's the evidence? Curr Med Res Opin 29(3):259–267

17. Patel TJ, Beredijklin BK, Matzon JL (2013) Trapeziometacarpal joint arthritis. Curr Rev Musculoskelet Med 6(1):1–8
18. Swindells MG, Logan AJ, Armstrong DJ, Chan P, Burke FD, Lindau TR (2010) The benefit of radiologically-guided steroid injections for trapeziometacarpal osteoarthritis. Ann R Coll Surg Engl 92:680–684
19. Hollander R (1951) The local effects of compound F [hydrocortisone] injected into joints. Bull Rheum Dis II(2):341–342
20. Snibbe JC, Gambardella RA (2005) Use of injections for osteoarthritis in joints and sports activity. Clin Sports Med 24(1):83–91
21. Roberts WN et al (1996) Corticosteroid injection in rheumatoid arthritis does not increase rate of total joint arthroplasty. J Rheumatol 23:1001–1004
22. Balazs EA, Denlinger JL (1993) Viscosupplementation: a new concept in the treatment of osteoarthritis. J Rheumatol Suppl 39:3–9
23. Altman RD (2003) Status of Hyaluronan supplementation therapy in osteoarthritis. Curr Rheumatol Rep 5:7–14
24. Abatangelo G, O'Regan M (1995) Hyaluronan: biological role and function in articular joints. Eur J Rheumatol Inflamm 15:9–16
25. Hiscock DDR, Caterson B, Flannery CR (2000) Expression of hyaluronan synthases in articular cartilage. Osteoarthr Cartil 8:120–126
26. Nishida Y, D'Souza AL, Thonar EJ, Knudson W (2000) Stimulation of hyaluronan metabolism by interleukin-1a in human articular cartilage. Arthritis Rheum 43:1315–1326
27. Takahashi K, Goomer RS, Harwood F et al (1999) The effects of hyaluronan on matrix metalloproteinase-3 (MMP-3), interleukin-1beta(IL-1beta), and tissue inhibitor of metalloproteinase-1 (TIMP-1) gene expression during the development of osteoarthritis. Osteoarthritis Cartilage 7:182–190
28. Asari A, Miyauchi S, Matsuzaka S et al (1998) Histomorphometric and biochemical effect of various hyaluronans on early osteoarthritis. J Rheumatol 25:1813–1819
29. Culty M, Miyake K, Kincade PW et al (1990) The hyaluronate receptor is a member of the CD44 (H-CAM) family of cell surface glycoproteins. J Cell Biol 111:2765–2774
30. Moreland LW (2003) Intra-articular hyaluronan (hyaluronic acid) and hylans for the treatment of osteoarthritis: mechanisms of action. Arthritis Res Ther 5:54–67
31. Punzi L (2001) The complexity of the mechanisms of action of hyaluronan in joint diseases. Clin Exp Rheumatol 19:242–246
32. Dahl LB, Dahl IM, Engstrom-Laurent A et al (1985) Concentration and molecular weight of sodium hyaluronate in synovial fluid from patients with rheumatoid arthritis and other arthropathies. Ann Rheum Dis 44:817–822
33. Castellacci E, Polieri T (2004) Antalgic effect and clinical tolerability of hyaluronic acid in patients with degenerative diseases of knee cartilage: an outpatient treatment survey. Drugs Exp Clin Res 30:67–73
34. Ghosh P, Guidolin D (2002) Potential mechanism of action of intra-articular hyaluronan therapy in osteoarthritis: are the effects molecular weight dependent? Semin Arthritis Rheum 32:10–37
35. Smith MM, Ghosh P (1987) The synthesis of hyaluronic acid by human synovial fibroblasts is influenced by the nature of the hyaluronate in the extracellular environment. Rheumatol Int 7:113–122
36. Vitanzo PC Jr, Sennett BJ (2006) Hyaluronans: is clinical effectiveness dependent on molecular weight? Am J Orthop 35:421–428
37. Roux C, Fontas E, Breuil V, Brocq O, Albert C, Euller-Ziegler L (2077) Injection of intra-articular sodium hyaluronidate (Sinovial) into the carpometacarpal joint of the thumb (CMC1) in osteoarthritis. A prospective evaluation of efficacy. Joint Bone Spine 74(4):368–372
38. Bahadir C, Onal B, Dayan VY, Gurer N (2009) Comparison of therapeutic effects of sodium hyaluronate and corticosteroid injections on trapeziometacarpal joint osteoarthritis. Clin Rheumatol 28(5):529–533

39. Fuchs S, Monikes R, Wohlmeiner A, Heyse T (2006) Intra-articolar hyaluronic acid compared with corticoid injections for the treatment of rhizarthrosis. Osteoarthr Cartil 14(1):82–88
40. Weiss S, LaStayo P, Mills A et al (2000) Prospective analysis of splinting the first carpometacarpal joint: an objective, subjective, and radiographic assessment. J Hand Ther 13:218–226
41. Swigart CR, Eaton RG, Glickel SZ, Johnson C (1999) Splinting in the treatment of arthritis of the first carpometacarpal joint. J Hand Surg Am 24A:86–91
42. Swigart CR (2008) Arthritis of the base of the thumb. Curr Rev Musculoskelet Med 1:142–146
43. Gomes Carreira AC, Jones A, Natour J (2010) Assessment of the effectiveness of a functional splint for osteoarthritis of the trapeziometacarpal joint of the dominant hand: a randomized controlled study. J Rehabil Med 42(5):469–474
44. Sillem H, Bockman CL, Miller WC, Li LC (2011) Comparison of two carpometacarpal stabilizing splints for individuals with thumb osteoarthritis. J Hand Ther 24(3):216–225
45. Bani MA, Arazpour M, Kashani RV, Mousavi ME, Hutchins SW (2013) Comparison of custom-made and prefabricated neoprene splinting in patients with the first carpometacarpal joint osteoarthritis. Disabil Rehabil Assist Technol 8(3):232–237
46. Weiss S, LaStayo P, Mills A, Bramlet D (2000) Splinting the first carpometacarpal joint: an objective, subjective, and radiographic assessment. J Hand Ther 13(3):218–235
47. Burke JH, Grady JH, de Vries J, Baten CTM (1999) Usability of thenar eminence orthoses: report a comparative study. Clin Rehabil 13(4):288–294
48. Neumann DA, Bielefeld T (2003) The carpometacarpal joint of the thumb: stability, deformity, and therapeutic intervention. J Orthop Sports Phys Ther 33:386–399
49. Hammond A, Freeman K (2001) One-year outcomes of a randomized controlled trial of an educational-behavioural joint protection programme for people with rheumatoid arthritis. Rheumatology 40:1044–1051
50. Pellegrini VD Jr (2001) Pathomechanics of the thumb trapeziometacarpal joint. Hand Clin 17:175–184
51. Valdes K, von der Heyde R (2012) An exercise program for carpometacarpal osteoarthritis based on biomechanical principles. J Hand Ther 25:251–263
52. Zhang W, Doherty M, Loed BF et al (2007) Eular evidence based recommendations for the management of hand osteoarthritis report of a task force of the Eular Standing Committee for international Clinical Studies Including Therapeutics (ESCISIT). Ann Rheum Dis 66:377–388
53. Rogers MW, Wilder FV (2009) Exercise and hand osteoarthritis symptomatology: a controlled crossover trial. J Hand Ther 22:10–18
54. Stamm TA, Machold KP, Smolen JS et al (2002) Joint protection and home hand exercises improve hand function in patients with hand osteoarthritis: a randomized controlled trial. Arthritis Rheum 47:44–49

5 Portals in the Arthroscopy of the Wrist and of the Small Joints

Arthroscopy of the wrist and small joints was born in the 1980s, although the first publication appeared in 1979 [1] and developed later in the 1990s. The European group of arthroscopy (EWAS—European Wrist Arthroscopy Society) was founded on 15 March 2005, by a group of friends who shared the same passion: Da Rin, Levadoux, Martinache, Rigault Mouton, Samson, Dumontier, Mathoulin, Moreel, Tchenio, Limousin, Cousin, Messina, Wilson, Amin, Fontes, Roure, Haerle and Lingo, Camps, with the collaboration of J. Dupuy (Storz). The first president of the group was Christian Dumontier and the first secretary Christophe Mathoulin [2]. Currently the members of the company are about 450 around the world, indicating that this technique is increasingly relevant in the wrist-hand surgery. The realization of increasingly small and sophisticated tools simplified the techniques and led to new endoscopic surgeries.

The system uses dedicated tools, such as optical ranging from 1 to 2.7 mm. They are positioned a 30° obliquity in order to get a broader view of the area. The optical fibre enters the trocar; together they have a length of 8–10 cm. It has two adjustable valves for the entry and exit of water. The motorized instruments have a thickness which spans from 1.2 to 2.7 mm. Not only the palpators are small in the apex—1/2 mm—but they are also short, in order to bring the hand of the operator close to the patient's, for better stability. Since we are working in such a small area, very few millimetres can change completely the field of view. Other tools dedicated to specific surgeries were gradually produced, such as baskets with straight, left or right blade, grippers and compasses to dig holes in the bone or to perform reductions of fractures or osteotomies (Fig. 5.1).

When we perform this technique, the patient is positioned supine on the operating table. The limb we must operate is lying on a table located on the side of the bed.

We normally use regional anaesthesia of the axillary plexus. Depending on the intervention, we eventually apply a tourniquet to the root of the limb.

After the sterile field is prepared, we apply a traction which can be vertical or horizontal, depending on the requirements:

S. Odella, *Trapeziometacarpal Joint Osteoarthritis*,
https://doi.org/10.1007/978-3-319-44336-2_5

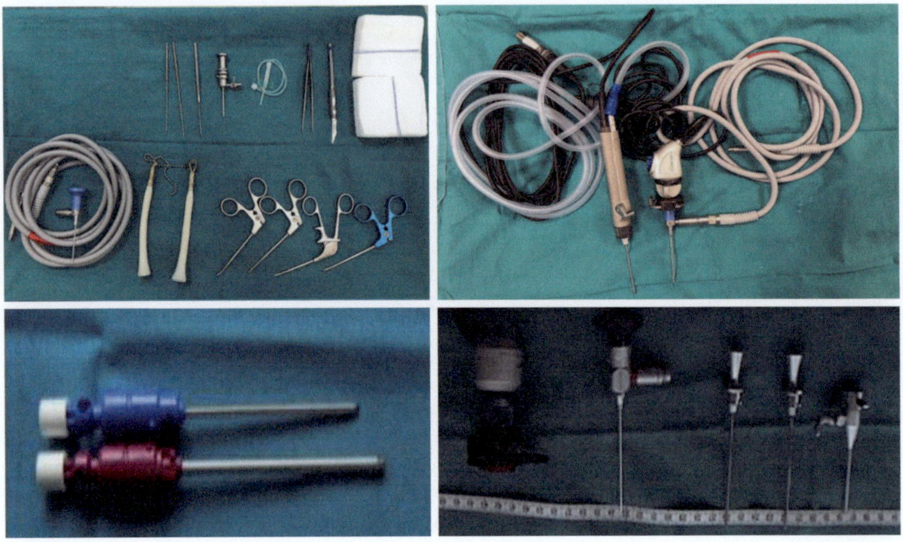

Fig. 5.1 The basic instruments used in arthroscopy. The camera has a controlled zoom and the possibility to adjust the brightness directly from the surgeon

- If the traction is vertical, the arm rests on the table, the elbow is flexed to 90° and the forearm and the hand are in a vertical position.
- If the traction is horizontal, the arm, forearm, wrist and hand are lying on the table along the same axis and the traction is fixed on the same table.

The pulling tower we use must have certain characteristics:

(a) It must be able to be used both horizontally and vertically.
(b) It should allow the evaluation of the traction with dynamometers.
(c) It should permit the use of X-rays and intraoperative arthroscopy.
(d) It must allow the forced and lasting flexion or extension of the wrist.
(e) It must allow the transition from pronation to supination and vice versa during surgery.
(f) It must be sterilizable.

In our practice, we used the pulley tower Borelli, which had all those characteristics.

Finger tractions are different in structure and material: those can be made of metal or plastic; the spatula-shaped traction can simultaneously grasp all the fingers of the hand, with an interlocking system.

The finger traps all have this same feature: they must tighten their finger during the traction and release them when the traction is removed; they also have to be sterile and sterilizable.

The traction is applied depending on the district that is going to be operated and on the pathology. For example, if you need to work on the thumb for a rhizo arthritis, the traction applies only to this finger. If you want to work on the wrist in all its completeness, the traction will be applied instead on the third and second finger of the hand. The tension also depends on what you must do. Considering the first example, for the thumb, a traction of 1.5 kg in a woman is enough, while for a man, it can even reach 3 kg. In the traction of the wrist, the tension can reach 6–8 kg, but not more than that. The weight of the traction also depends on the duration of the operation.

Normally we use a saline solution that can be injected with or without the pump, normally with gravitational drop. Some operators do not use water, especially in the recent wrist fractures, because the water could expand between the fracture lines. We typically make the first reconnaissance without water. Eventually, by opening and closing the valve of the trocar, we can regulate the flow and pressure.

There are also some tools which are prepared before starting the operation. They are both motorized and radio-frequency devices, both of which have a small size and are specifically made for this type of technique. Needles are also prepared and can be used for minor repairs. Finally, small, curved Klemmer can be used to open the arthroscopic access.

So, once you established where to apply the traction—depending on the pathology to be treated—and how much weight you can apply to the fingers, you can proceed with the surgery.

This technique can be used in several ways:

(a) As a diagnostic
(b) As intra-articular surgery (removing movable bodies, repairing TFCs, etc.)
(c) As an aid to external surgery [3, 4]

It is necessary to establish the anatomic landmarks. Especially at the beginning, it is recommended to draw the landmarks; this can be done with the traction applied. If they are drawn without, they can be changed once the traction is in position.

The most used portal is the 3/4. We begin by drawing Lister's tubercle: a bone crest placed on the transition area between the long thumb extender and long radial extensor of the carpus. Once the tubercle is located, placing the thumb transversely on this structure, we can distally incise the skin. We can incise transversally, which is more aesthetic or we can incise vertically, which allows near-distal corrections or vice versa, in case the joint is not well-centred. Before the incision, we can reach with a needle the articular space and inject water. The water, by widening the joint, will favour the entry of the arthroscopic trocar (Fig. 5.2).

The entrance follows certain rules, which are shown in Fig. 5.3.

Portals are different and they all have a function, depending on what you need to see and what you need to do. Some portals allow the optical fibre vision, while others allow the entrance with appropriate tools and to perform the designed operation. We will now analyse every portal, and for each one, we will describe what can be seen in the condition of anatomical normality. As you will see, they are named referring to the nearby anatomical structures, especially tendons. It should be considered that these portals are interchangeable between optic fibre and instrumentation and are used for both [5]. For the description of the ligaments, you can refer to (Fig. 5.4).

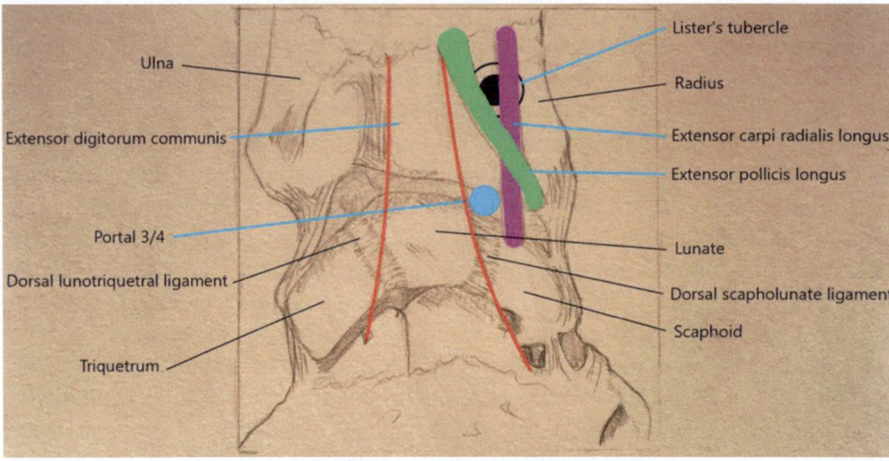

Fig. 5.2 We can see portal 3/4, distally from Lister's tubercle. (Adapted with permission from Adravanti P, Denti M, Mazzola C, Randelli P, Zorzi C. Artroscopia Base ed Avanzata. Rome: CIC Edizioni Internazionali)

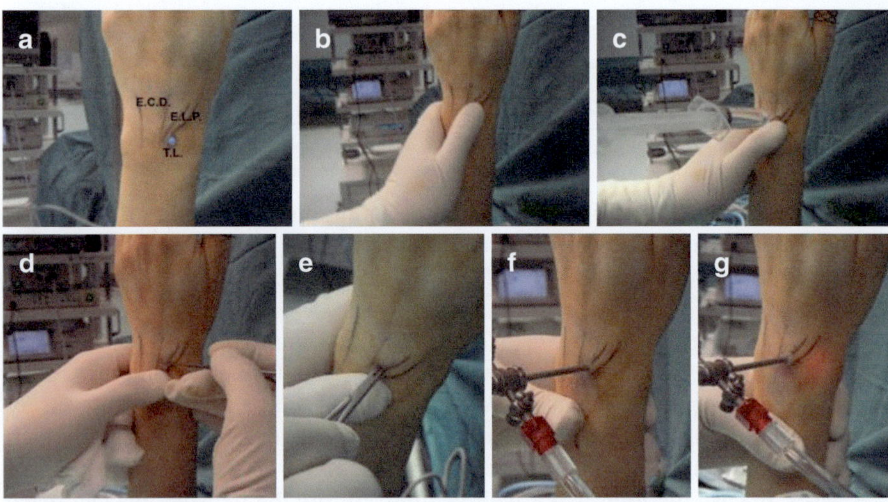

Fig. 5.3 The arthroscopic introduction in the radio-carpal through portal 3/4. (**a**) The first step is to locate Lister's tubercle (TL), the extensor digitorum communis (EDC) and the extensor pollicis longus (EPL). (**b**) We lean with the thumb on the tubercle and, 1–1.5 cm distally, we locate the articular space of the portal 3/4. (**c**) It is possible, especially at the beginning, to use a guide needle with water, which helps to open wide the joint. (**d**) Incision of the skin, in this case transversely. (**e**) Entrance with a curved Klemmer which is best suited to go around the epiphysis of the radius. (**f**) At this point we enter with the trocar and, leaving the sheath, (**g**) we enter with the arthroscope. (Reproduced with permission from Adravanti P, Denti M, Mazzola C, Randelli P, Zorzi C. Artroscopia Base ed Avanzata. Rome: CIC Edizioni Internazionali)

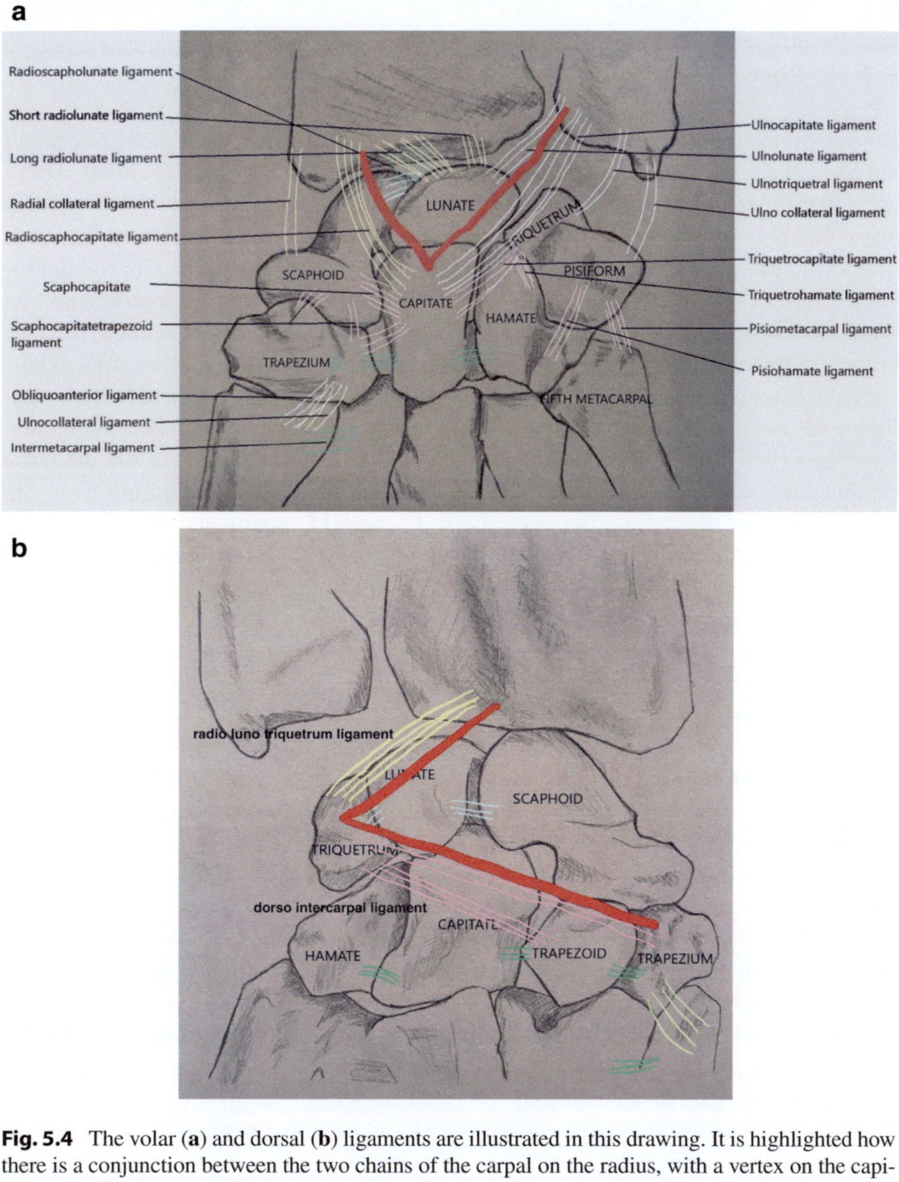

Fig. 5.4 The volar (**a**) and dorsal (**b**) ligaments are illustrated in this drawing. It is highlighted how there is a conjunction between the two chains of the carpal on the radius, with a vertex on the capitate. Dorsally the connection is between the radius and triquetrum with passing on the lunate. There is a ligament that, from the triquetrum, crosses transversally all the carpal bones; the vertex is precisely on the triquetrum. All of it is for a complete stability of the radio-ulnar-carpal ensemble. (Adapted with permission from Adravanti P, Denti M, Mazzola C, Randelli P, Zorzi C. Artroscopia Base ed Avanzata. Rome: CIC Edizioni Internazionali)

5.1 Dorsal Portals

5.1.1 Portal 1/2

By this portal we can access the radio-carpal joint radially. It then passes between the first (AbLP and EBP) and the second (ERCL and ERCB) dorsal channels. There are some precautions to locate it: we must remember that the styloid is raised to about 10° between the two radial and ulnar limits; therefore we are not on the same line as the portal 3/4, but somewhat more distal. We also must consider the dorso-volar angle of about 15° to position the arthroscope. We are in an anatomical area that presents the radial artery that leads to the anatomical snuffbox and the sensory branch of the radial nerve. It is therefore advisable to stay close to the carpal extensors. We can observe the scaphoid up to its distal recess, the styloid and radio-carpal ligaments radial from the styloid. In front of us we see the radius-scaphoid-capitate ligaments (RSC), the long radio-lunate ligament (RLL) and, closer to the ulna, the radius-scaphoid-lunate ligament (RSL or ligament of Testut) originating from the anterior limit of the radius. Between the RSC and RLL ligaments, there is a space which is often the origin of the cysts of the pulse. Beyond this space we meet the carpal flexion tendon (FCR). By turning the optic fibre, you can see all the radio-carpal dorsal capsules.

5.1.2 Portal 3/4

It is the most used portal because of its central position into the wrist. This gives us a good overview for the initial evaluation of the radio-carpal. This portal is thus accessed in the beginning of wrist arthroscopy.

Once entered, we face the long radius-scaphoid-lunate ligament (RSL) or ligament of Testut. The ligament continues with the scaphoid-lunate ligament in its volar part. From here with the palpator, we can test its endurance. We can also note the crest which separates the scaffold of radius from the semilunate of the radius. In the direction of the radius, we will see the same ligaments we saw in portal 1/2 and the radial face of the scaphoid. Moving in the direction of the ulna, on the volar side, we meet the short radiolunate ligament (RLC). This ligament has an oblique radial part which forms an inverted "V" with the RLL. The apex of the V—still in the volar part—meets the scaphoid-lunate (SL). Continuing in the ulnar side, we see the triangular ligament with some of its components:

- The insertion on the radius: it's difficult to see with the optical fibre, although you can palpate it.
- The palmar radio-ulnar ligament: it's the main stabilizer of the triangular ligament on the volar side.

Then we see the ulno-lunate (UL) and ulno-triquetrum (UT) ligaments. Between the two of them, we should be able to identify the ligament ulno-triquetrum-capitate

(UPC), also called ulno-capitate (UC). It forms a “V” with the ligament RSC. On the apex of the “V”, there is the capitate. The two of them stabilize the two chains in the volar side. The UPC ligament seems to be a more superficial reinforcement than the ligament UP. Therefore, it is not visible from the inside of the joint. We can see the carpal surface of the pyramid until the prestyloid recess and the interosseous luno-triquetrum ligament. This also must be palpated to test its stability.

5.1.3 Portal 4/5

This portal is placed between the extensor digitorum (ED) and the extensor digiti minimi (EDM). This is usually a small space. It is therefore advisable to stick to the ulnar margin of the ED, because it is the most evident upon palpation. This is not particularly difficult; the intra-articular vision is better in the ulnar sector. We will have a good view of the insertion of the triangular ligament on the radius and of the ligaments and bone surfaces we saw in the compartment 3/4. By turning the optic fibre, we can observe the dorsal part of scaphoid-lunate and its continuity on the dorsal capsule. Pushing the optic fibre a little to the volar direction, you can get to the pisiform-triquetral articulation and pre-styloid ulnar recesses.

5.1.4 Portal 6R

This portal is located on the radius side of the tendon of extensor carpi ulnaris (ECU). It is placed distally to the triangular ligament. Therefore, the reference for the entry point is the ulnar styloid, not the epiphyseal edge of the ulna. With this portal, we can observe very well:

- The triangular ligament in all its length, the UL and UP ligaments.
- The pre-styloid recesses and pisiform-triquetral articulation can be viewed in their entirety.
- The semilunar fossa of the radius.
- The surface of the lunate and of the triquetrum up to the distal ulnar apex.
- The ulnocarpal ligaments
- The interosseous luno-triquetral ligament.
- Also, by lowering proximally, we can see the space below the triangular ligament, between the caput ulnae and the triangular ligament.

5.1.5 Portal 6U

This portal is placed ulnarly compared to the ECU tendon. It presents the risk of damaging the ulnar dorsal sensory nerve which passes near this entrance. It is therefore advisable to stay adherent to the tendon. This practice does not eliminate completely the risk of iatrogenic injury. Then, it is also advisable to make an incision of 1 cm, staying more superficially than the tendon. After that we will divaricate with a chamfer tool the skin until we reach the vicinity of the tendon. Only then we will use the trocar to enter the joint. The part we can better observe with this entry is the triangular ligament. It is also visible in its dorsal part with the radio-ulnar distal dorsal ligament (RUDD) and the radio-ulnar distal palmar ligament. They both lead to the fovea at the base of the ulnar styloid and give stability to the distal radio-ulnar joint.

5.2 Medio-carpal Radial (MCR) Portal

This portal is located approximately 1 cm distally from the portal 3/4. It forms an angle with the horizontal, from top to bottom and from dorsal to volar, of about 15°. In addition, the range of extensors tends to widen distally. Therefore, if we climb vertically from the portal 3/4, we can damage the tendon of the second finger of the extensor digitorum. It is therefore advisable to take as a reference the metacarpal phalngeal (MF) of the second finger and draw a line with the entry of the portal 3/4. We must then palpate the tendon and, keeping ourselves close to it, penetrate the joint. We are now in the medio-carpal, in the space between the scaphoid and lunate, above the round face of the capitate. In front of us there is the RSC ligament. Ulnarly we can observe the distal face of the lunate, the space between the lunate and triquetrum and the distal articular surface of the triquetrum. By moving distally around the proximal pole of the capitate and volarly from the UPC ligament, we are able to identify the articulation between the triquetrum and hamate. From the radial side, we can see the entire distal surface of the scaphoid until the scaphoid-trapezium-trapezoid (STT).

5.2.1 Midcarpal Ulnar Portal (MCU)

The portal is placed at 1–1.5 cm distally from the portal 4/5. We will perform the same operation we did for MCR portal. This time we will mark the line which connects the entrance point 4/5 with the epiphysis of the fifth metacarpal in a depression between the trapezium and the hamate. The direction is the same: inclined from dorsal to volar and from distal to proximal of about 15°. We are at the meeting of the four defined corners for the arthrodesis (four corners). It is more difficult to see the STT. We can see instead the distal articular surface of the trapezium, the semilunar and the scaphoid. We can also see so the interposed ligaments (scaphoid-lunate and triquetrum-lunate). Distally we can follow the proximal pole of the capitate. Volarly we identify the UPC ligaments in the portion triquetrum-capitate, which meet in the inverted "V" with the RSC. We can see the space between the triquetrum, the semilunar, the capitate and the hamate, until the hook of the hamate.

5.2.2 Anterior Portals

Recently, surgeons have developed volar portals to view the articulation from palmar to dorsal, especially to see in full the S-L and L-P ligaments in their entirety.

We can also use them to see dorsal ligaments and for some surgeries. Volar portals have also been used for a long time in case of repair of wrist fractures with the use of volar plaques. In this case the access did not require any caution, being open-air surgery.

5.2.3 Volar Radial Portal (VR)

This is a portal which has been used recently and is performed, according to Slutsky [6], by incising the skin over the FCR tendon. Then, once located, we move it either medially or laterally, and we access below the tendon itself. We prefer to access in another way: before surgery, if we want a volar access, by using the Doppler scan, we locate the radial artery and mark it on the skin. We mark, then, the FCR tendon. We prepare the traction, and through the portal 3/4, we locate the space between the RSC and RLL and we place the optic fibre in the established point. We remove the optics leaving the trocar sheath, with a switching stick we enter the sheath and, with the optic placed on another radio-carpal portal, we observe. We push the stick ulnarly to the FCR tendon, which is usually the safest passage (Fig. 5.5). With this portal, we can see the scaphoid-lunate ligament in its front portion and the triquetrum-lunate with all the carpal bone surfaces of the scaphoid and of the semilunar. The triquetrum vision is a bit more difficult, because there is the pisiform which blocks the motility of the optic fibre. We can see the articular surface of the radius, with the crest and the two articular faces: one for the scaphoid and one for the lunate, the radio-lunate-triquetrum (RLP) ligament. We can also see the triangular ligament in its insertion on the radius with its inferior radial lateral ligament (RUID), which is the other stabilizing component of the triangular ligament.

5.2.4 Ulnar Volar Portal (VU)

The entrance technique is the same as the in-out, but this time the landmark is the tendon of the flexor carpi ulnaris (FCU), the ulnar artery and the ulnar nerve. Another landmark is the pisiform. Slutsky [7], on the other hand, uses a more medial approach by using the flexor digitorum superficialis as a reference point: once isolated and moved radially, he passes behind it, thus entering the articulation. With this portal, we see better the ulnar compartment, especially the LP ligament.

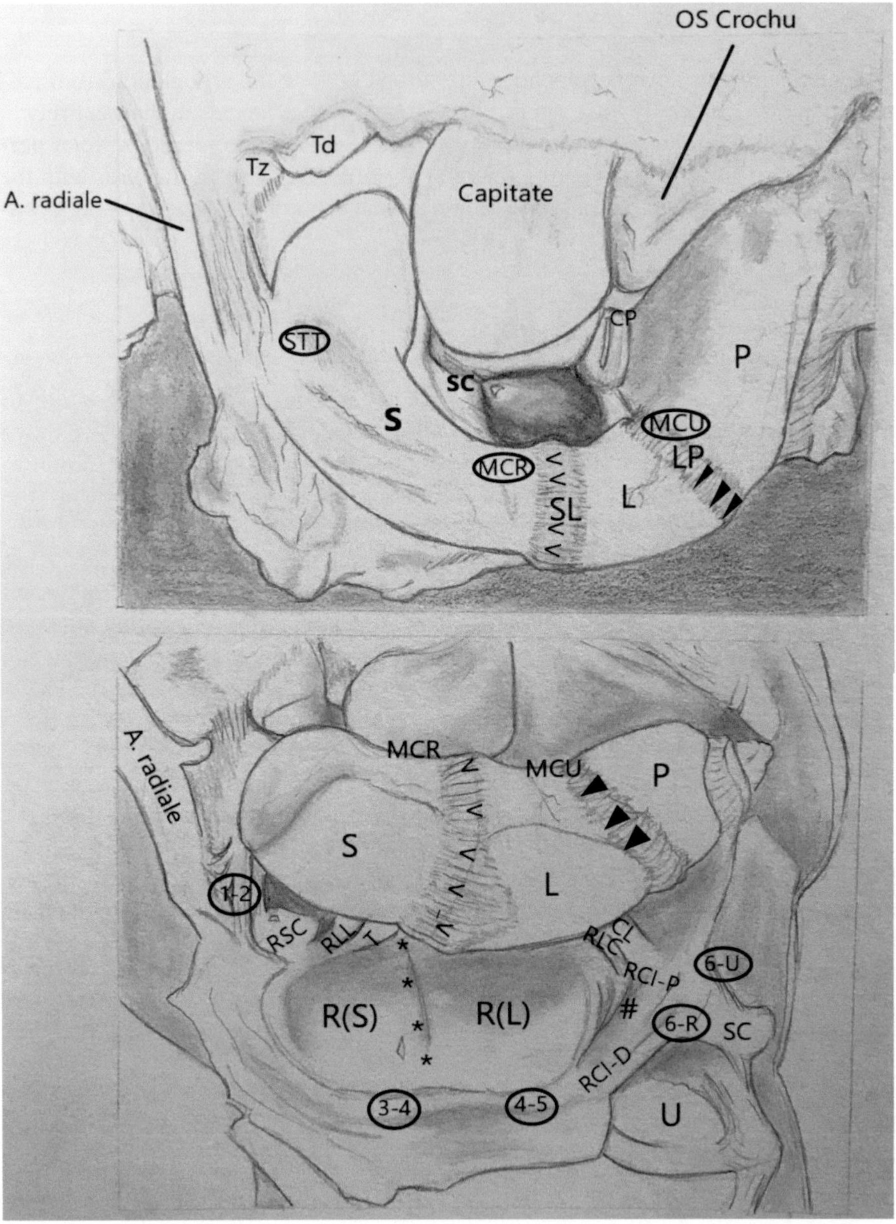

Fig. 5.5 In this anatomic cross-section the structures and portals are reported, in A of the radio-ulno-carpic and in B the medium-carpic. The portals of the trapezium-metacarpal, the distal radio-ulnar and the radio-ulno-carpal portal are not reported here. The pisiforme is not evident. (Adopted from Atzei A, Luchetti R, Sgarbossa A, Carità E, Llusàc M. Installation, voies d'abord et exploration normale en arthroscopie du poignet. Chirurgie de la Main. 2006;25:S131–44)

5.3 Portals to STT

5.3.1 STT Portal

We should immediately point out that, in this case, the traction is applied only to the thumb and usually consists of 2–3 kg. It depends on the subject, age and articular condition. Until now we have seen the radio-carpal and intercarpal portals. Now we will see the access portals to STT. The STT-U portal is into the space at the apex of the scaphoid. We must pay attention to the presence of the radial artery and the radial nerve sensory branch. Usually, we use the MCR portal and we move to the apex of the scaphoid. Then we palpate and see with the optics where we are palpating; this way we can understand our external position and introduce a needle. Also in this case, with a preoperative Doppler scan, we can draw the artery on the skin. It is also useful to draw the tendons of extensor pollicis longus (EPL) and extensor pollicis brevis (EBP). Once entered, with the trocar we switch the optics: in this space, we see the distal pole of the scaphoid, the proximal articular surface of the trapezium and the trapezoid. If we must work here, it is useful to use the optics in the MCR portal and the tools in the STT portal. Otherwise we can access from a more volar portal at the base of the thenar, called STT-R portal [8].

5.4 Trapezium-Metacarpal Portals

5.4.1 Trapezium-Metacarpal Radial Portal (TMR, Also Called 1R)

This portal is located radially to the longitudinal axis of the abductor pollicis longus. It allows to view the distal surface of the trapezium, the proximal surface of the metacarpal, the dorsal radial ligaments (DR), posterior oblique ligament (LPO) and ulnar collateral ligament (UCL).

5.4.2 Trapezoidal-Metacarpal-Ulnar Portal (TMU, Also Called 1U)

This portal is located either between the tendon of EPL and EBP or ulnarly to EPL. The radial artery is very close to the portal. In order to avoid it, it is advisable to stay closer to EBP. It shows, as for the 1R portal, the articulations described. We can see them, unlike the 1R, from an ulnar-radial view. The anterior oblique ligament (AOL) and the ulnar collateral ligament (UCL) are highlighted.

There are two more portals which favour a vision of the dorsal portion of this articulation. One is the Orellana portal, bearing the name of the one who used it first, presented in 2003. It is placed more radially and before the 1R, and it is also called 2R. The other was developed by Slutsky in 2007. It passes between the first and second metacarpals and reaches the trapezium-metacarpal, highlighting the dorsal surface of this articulation and the carpal ligament. It is called 2D.

5.5 Radio-ulnar Distal (RUD) Articulation Portals [9, 10]

Returning dorsally, we can use some portals to highlight the radio-ulnar distal articulation. It is raising increasingly more interest because of the evaluation of the stability and because of the view of the triangular ligament from the proximal part and the sigmoidal articulation.

5.5.1 Radio-ulnar Distal Lower (RUDL) Portal

This portal is identified by looking for the articulation between the radius and ulna. It is placed at about 0.5–1 cm from the 6R portal, slightly more radicalized. If finding it proves difficult, we can use the portal 3/4. We palpate the end of the triangular ligament on its insertion to the radio. Below there is the Distal radio-ulnar joint (RUD) at 0.5, which is the thickness of the triangular ligament. With this portal, we can see the proximal part of the triangular ligament, the entire articulation surface of the epiphysis and the insertion into the fovea of the deep part of the triangular ligament. From the radial side, we can see the sigmoid depression of the radius. A practical aspect should be considered: a vertical traction is useful to view the deep part of the triangular ligament; too much traction, on the other side, closes the distal radio-ulnar joint.

5.5.2 Proximal Lower Radio-ulnar Portal (PLRUP)

This portal is about 1–1.5 cm below the RUDL portal, on the same direction. It is used to work on the RUD articulation, between RUID and RUIP. It views the proximal part of caput ulnae and the proximal face of the sigmoid radial surface. In conclusion, it views the RUD articulation, more proximally.

References

1. Chen YC (1979) Arthroscopic of the wrist and finger joints. Orthop Clin North Am 10:723–733
2. Mathoulin C, Levadoux M, Martinache X (2005) Intéreèt thérapeutique de l'arthroscopie du poignet: à propos de 1000 cas. e-mémoires de l'Académie Nationale de. Chirurgie 4(3):42–57
3. Del Pinal F, Mathoulin C, Luchetti R (2010) Arthroscopic management of distal radius fractures. Springer, Berlin
4. Da Rin F (2008) Il trattamento delle fratture del polso con assistenza artroscopia. Lo Scalpello 22:114–120
5. Abrams RA, Petersen M, Botte MJ (1994) Arthroscopic portals of the wrist: an anatomic study. J Hand Surg Am 19(6):940–944
6. Slutsky DJ (2002) Wrist arthroscopy through a volar radial portal. Arthroscopy 18(6):624–630
7. Slutsky DJ (2004) The use of a volar ulnar portal in wrist arthroscopy. Arthroscopy 20(2):158–163

8. Mathoulin C, Da Rin F (2011) Arthroscopic treatment of Scaphotrapeziotrapezoid Osteoarthritis In: Slutsky DJ (Guest ed) New advances in wrist and small joint arthroscopy. Hand clinics, vol 27, no 3, pp 319–322
9. Luchetti R, Da Rin F, Borelli PP, Mathoulin C, Atzei A, Khanchandani P (2008) Arthroscopically assisted Sauvè-Kapandji procedure: an advanced technique for distal radioulnar joint arthritis. Tech Hand Up Extrem Surg 12(4):216–220
10. Berger RA (1999) Arthroscopic anatomy of the wrist and distal radioulnar joint. Hand Clin 15(3):393–413

Trapeziometacarpal Joint Arthrosis: Arthroscopic Treatment

6

Osteoarthritis of the first column relates to the trapeziometacarpal and the trapezium-trapezoid-hull acme (STT). The two neighbouring joints work together. This relation can modify, in a consistent way, the surgical decision. Therefore, we divided into two parts the treatment of the two diseases, but we presented some of the contact points between them, both in the surgical technique and in the context of the disease itself.

6.1 The Trapeziometacarpal Joint Arthrosis

The introduction in the market of small and technological optical devices allowed the surgeon to access and operate even the smallest joints.

This has led to the development, in 1995, of the trapeziometacarpal joint arthroscopy [1, 2].

The arthroscopy allowed the surgeon to work within the joint without altering its stability and accelerated the recovery of the motility.

Clearly, the passage from arthroscopy to open surgery must always be possible.

6.2 Anatomy of the Trapeziometacarpal Joint [3]

The joint has a concave-convex geometric shape which allows the movement even with a significant translation of the two surfaces of the joint.

The ligaments and the capsule have a particular arrangement: they split into a complex ulno-volar, dorsoradial and in an intermetacarpal ligament.

S. Odella, *Trapeziometacarpal Joint Osteoarthritis*,
https://doi.org/10.1007/978-3-319-44336-2_6

The most important ligaments are four (Pictures 6.1 and 6.2):

1. The dorsoradial ligament (Arnold external trapezium-metacarpal)
2. The dorsal-ulnar ligament (Arnold trapezium-internal metacarpal) or posterior oblique
3. The anterior oblique ligament
4. The intermetacarpal ligament

The damage of one of them may cause instability.

In the joint we also have the metacarpal *abductor pollicis longus* insertion and the segment of the trapeziometacarpal *extensor pollicis brevis* and *longus* in the dorsal part of the joint.

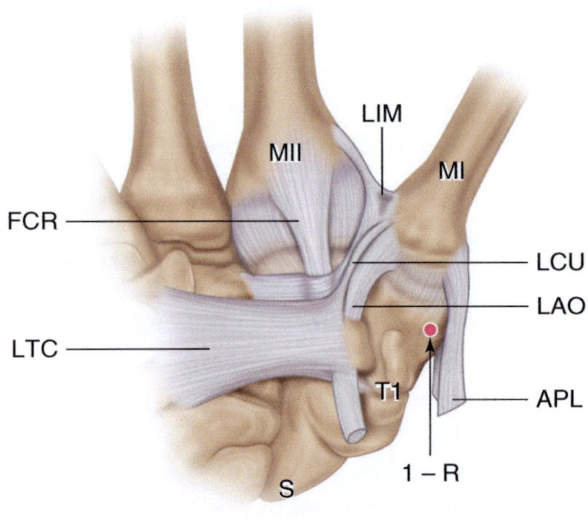

Picture 6.1 Dyagram of TM ligaments. *AOL* Anterior oblique ligament, *UCL* ulnar collateral ligament, *IML* intermetacarpal ligament, *APL* abductor pollicis Longus, *T1* trapezium, *M1* 1st metacarpus, *MII* 2nd metacarpus, *S* scaphoid, *TCL* transverse ligament of the carpus, 1-R portal. Image from the book "Wrist arthroscopy" R. Luchetti; A.Atzei Ed.Mattioli 2001

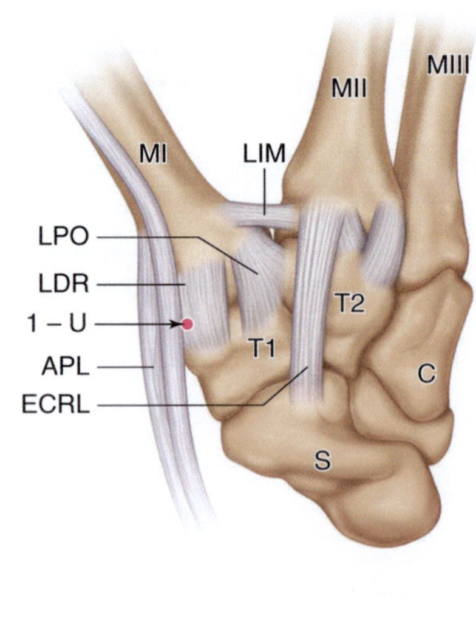

Picture 6.2 Diagram of dorsal vision of TM ligaments. *POL* posterior oblique ligament, *DRL* dorso-radial ligament, *IML* intermetacarpal ligament, *ERCL* long radial extensor, *APL* abductor pollicis Longus, *T1* trapezius, *T2* trapezoid, *M1* 1st metacarpus, *MII* 2nd metacarpus, *MIII* 3° metacarpus, *S* scaphoid, *1-U* ulnar portal from the book "Arthroscopy of the wrist" R. Luchetti; A.Atzei Ed.Mattioli 2001

Other anatomical elements that must be considered are:

1. The deep and superficial branch of the radial artery
2. The nerve branches of the forearm lateral cutaneous nerve terminals
3. The sensory branches of the radial nerve

All those elements are very close to the articulation itself.

6.3 Classification

The rhizarthrosis was classified according to the radiographic appearance of Eaton-Glickel in 1987 (Picture 6.1, Fig. 6.1):

Stage 1: initial reduction of the interarticular space and osteosclerosis of the borders, possibly with initial osteophytes, especially on the trapezoid
Stage 2: advanced reduction the interarticular space. Initial peritrapezial osteoarthritis
Stage 3: initial subluxation of the trapeziometacarpal and adduction of metacarpal

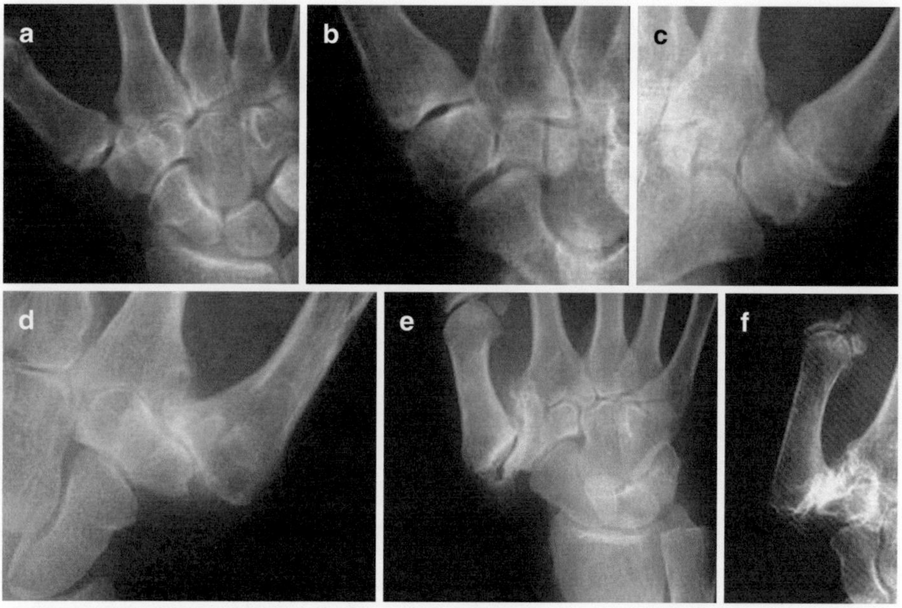

Fig. 6.1 The rhizarthrosis radiographic classification of Eaton-Glickel in 1987. (**a**) Stage 1: initial reduction of the interarticular space and osteosclerosis of the borders, possibly with initial osteophytes, especially on the trapezoid. (**b**) Stage 2: advanced reduction the interarticular space. Initial peritrapezial osteoarthritis. (**c**) Stage 3: initial subluxation of the trapeziometacarpal and adduction of metacarpal. (**d**) Stage 4: severe osteoarthritis of the trapezium-metacarpal and peritrapezial with fixed adduction metacarpal. Subluxation >1/3 of the trapeziometacarpal. (Reproduced with permission from Adravanti P, Denti M, Mazzola C, Randelli P, Zorzi C. Artroscopia Base ed Avanzata. Rome: CIC Edizioni Internazionali)

Stage 4: severe osteoarthritis of the trapezium-metacarpal and peritrapezial with fixed adduction metacarpal Subluxation > 1/3 of the trapeziometacarpal

Mennon made a classification that also evaluated the clinical aspect associated with radiographic appearance:

Stage 1: pain at the base of the thumb, no deformity and crepitus during the movement

Reduction of the joint space, marginal osteophytes

Stage 2: pain and crepitus. Significant reduction of the articular space, cysts of the metacarpal or trapeze, sclerosis, minimum subluxation of the metacarpal, normality of the metacarpophalangeal and the first space

Step 3: Step 2 + 1/3 subluxation of the base of the metacarpal, hyperextension of the metacarpophalangeal >10°

Stage 4:

(a) Stage 3 + subluxation of the base of the metacarpal >1/3, hyperextension of the metacarpophalangeal >10°, adduction of the metacarpal with preserved mobility

(b) Fixity metacarpal adduction (no preservation of the mobility)

Stage 5: osteoarthritis of the TM + osteoarthritis of the STT

Dr. Badia from Miami presented, in the occasion of the meeting on rhizarthrosis in Cortina (2002), an arthroscopic classification and its treatment, according to the following stages [4]:

Stage I: diffuse synovitis without damage of the cartilage or the presence of a small lesion associated with a ligamentous laxity of the palmar capsular part (arthroscopic synovectomy)

Stage II: lesion of the cartilage of the trapezium associated to ligamentous laxity; presence, sometimes, of a movable body (synovectomy, shrinkage, removal of any movable body osteotomy and Wilson)

Stage III: cartilage injury of the trapezoid and the base of the first metacarpal (hemi resection of arthroscopic trapezium with interposition)

6.4 Surgical Technique Brief

The access to the trapeze-metacarpal is the subject of another chapter of the monograph.

The landmarks are the bone contours of the two joint components and the tendon of *adductor longus* and *extensor pollicis brevis*. If we need to be more precise, we can follow the radial artery with a Doppler scan before applying the tourniquet and perform the procedure. We must always remember that the anatomical location may vary with traction (Picture 6.2, Fig. 6.2).

In order to insert the arthroscope, we must get the right diastasis of the joint, which is 90°. To achieve that, we will apply a traction of 2 kg to the thumb and a counter traction at the elbow [6, 7].

The two portals are 1R and 1U. They are placed on either side of the tendons of *abductor pollicis longus* (Ab.L), *extensor pollicis brevis* (E.B.P.) and *extensor pollicis longus* (E.L.P.) (Pictures 6.1 and 6.2).

First, we introduce a needle 20 in any of the two portals (depending on the surgeon) and inject 2dc of water. We will then cut the skin with a blade 15 and, with a chamfer tool, widen the access. After that we introduce the trocar, which presents a useful graph marking, and then the 1.9 mm optical. In the other portals is usually introduced the motorized tool with drills 2.2 (Fig. 6.3) or the apparatus of the radio frequency (Fig. 6.4) in order to observe the arthroscopic surgery. With the abrader ball, we resect the articular portion of the trapezium by a few millimetres (Figs. 6.3 and 6.4).

Subsequently we insert a spacer which can be made with artificial, resorbable material—like Artelon®—or biological material such as *palmar gracilis* in which it is wounded on itself like an anchovy (Fig. 6.5).

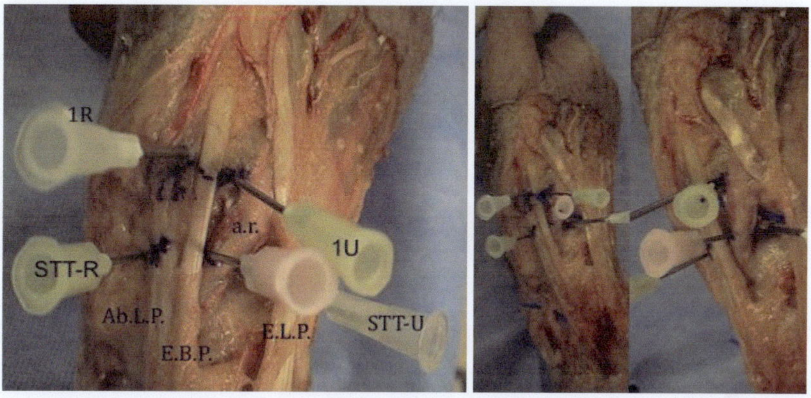

Fig. 6.2 Anatomical aspect: radial artery (ar), tendon of long abductor (AbLP). The tendon of extensor pollicis brevis (EBP) and of extensor pollicis longus (ELP). The trapezium-metacarpal (TM) access portals are 1R and 1U. There is a more volar portal identified by Orellana which is the 2R and another portal described by Slutsky [5] which is the 2D. For the scaphoid-trapezium-trapezoid (STT), the portals are STT-U and STT-R. (Reproduced with permission from Adravanti P, Denti M, Mazzola C, Randelli P, Zorzi C. Artroscopia Base ed Avanzata. Rome: CIC Edizioni Internazionali)

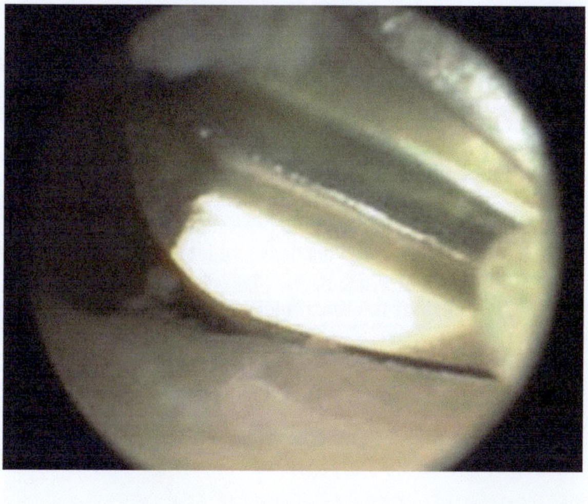

Fig. 6.3 The entrance of the motorized tool to resect the distal portion of the trapezium and facilitate the interposing of the spacer

The arthroscopy of the STT is also performed, in order to verify whether the trapezoid-scaphoid articulation is undamaged. If it is compromised, there are two solutions:

- The removal of the trapezium and making a suspension of the Weilby plastic [8, 9]
- The resection of the distal epiphysis of the scaphoid and the eventual application of a spacer

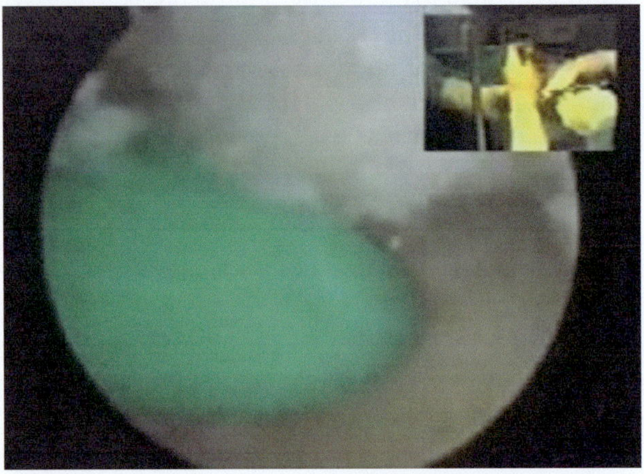

Fig 6.4 Use of radio frequencies to clean up the articulation from synovitis and/or to perform ligaments shrinkage

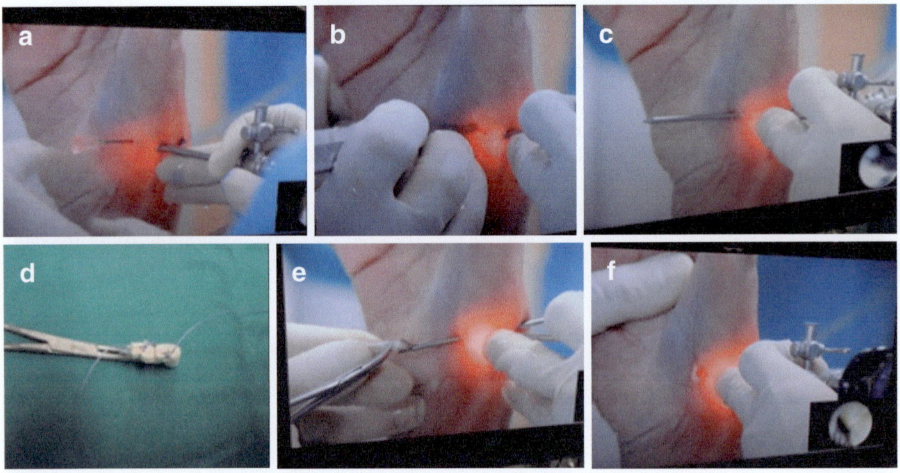

Fig. 6.5 The in-out technique for the spacer grip. In this case of the reabsorbable material, we locate the portal 2R (**a**), pass with the switching stick (**c**) after incising the skin (**b**) and come out of the articulation. We pass along the same way with a clamp (**e**), take the spacer (**d**) and drag it into the joint (**f**). Each step is always under the control of the optic fibre. (Reproduced with permission from Adravanti P, Denti M, Mazzola C, Randelli P, Zorzi C. Artroscopia Base ed Avanzata. Rome: CIC Edizioni Internazionali)

6.5 Errors and Complications

Injuries of radial artery, radial nerve branches and tendon of abductor longus have been described.

Even technical mistakes can occur as the creation of Intrauma-articulate mobile bodies or an insufficient resection that can cause impingement and pain (Figs. 6.6 and 6.7).

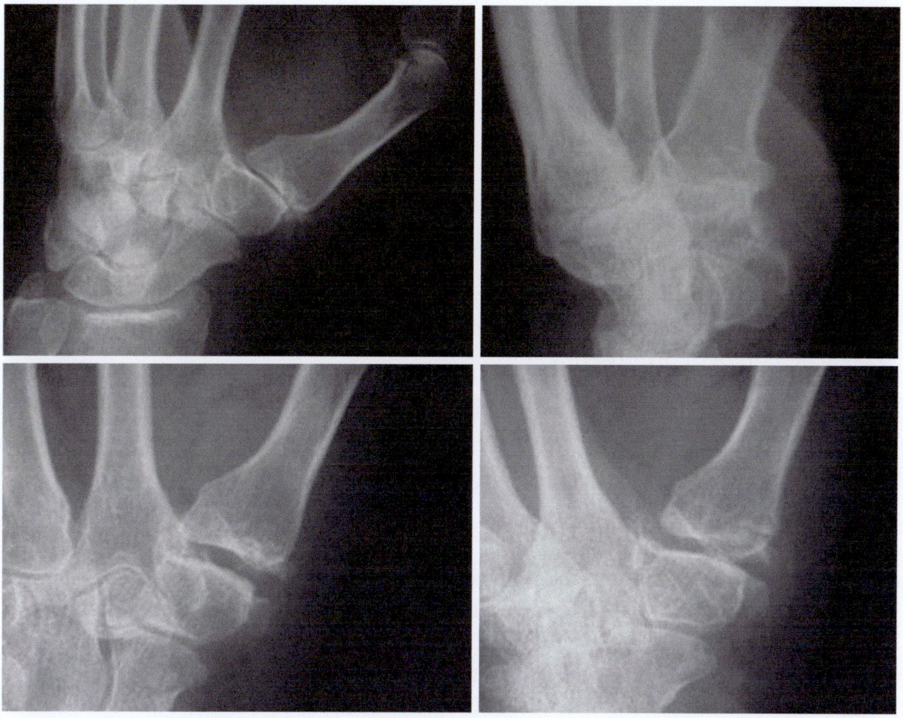

Fig. 6.6 Resective failure with the creation of endoarticular mobile bodies, which creates an impingement. (Reproduced with permission from Adravanti P, Denti M, Mazzola C, Randelli P, Zorzi C. Artroscopia Base ed Avanzata. Rome: CIC Edizioni Internazionali)

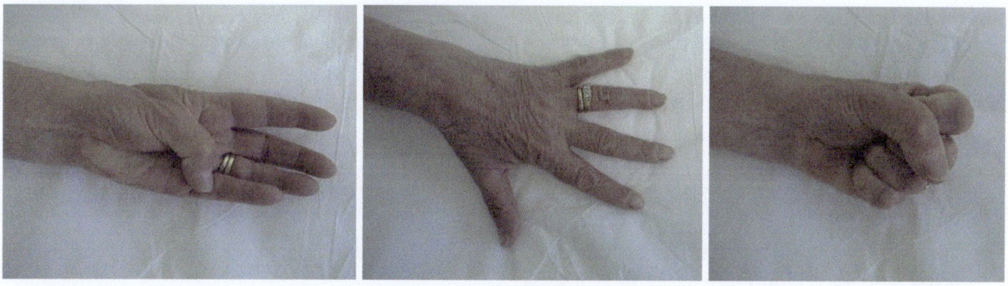

Fig. 6.7 Woman patient with distortive trauma and trapezium-metacarpal bone separation. Insufficient resection error with painful contact of the volar portion of the articulation. (Reproduced with permission from Adravanti P, Denti M, Mazzola C, Randelli P, Zorzi C. Artroscopia Base ed Avanzata. Rome: CIC Edizioni Internazionali)

Conclusions

The advantages of arthroscopic resection are:

1. No need of stabilizing plastic
2. Real evaluation of peritrapezial arthrosis and possibly to switch to open surgery for treatment
3. Highlighting of other associated lesions
4. Reduced immobilization times of about 12–21 days

The disadvantages are:

1. The difficulty of the technique
2. The necessity of a dedicated instrumentation
3. The cost

Contraindications to surgical arthroscopy:

1. The presence of trapezium-scaphoid and peritrapezial arthrosis
2. Instability of the trapezium-metacarpal
3. The failure of arthroscopy
4. Rigid thumb adduction
5. Rheumatoid arthritis
6. Metacarpus subluxation
7. Arthrosis degeneration in Eaton stage 4

Arthroscopy has given new surgical perspectives that will allow interventions which today are considered impossible to perform with this technique. But an even more important issue is the ability to recognize pathologies that instrumental examinations cannot highlight.

Another advantage is the ability to perform dynamic manoeuvres that allow to highlight the motility of articular structures during stress. It must always be considered the fact that you can at any times switch to open surgery.

References

1. Berger RA (1996) Arthroscopic of the 1st CMC (trapeziometacarpal) Joint. AAOS Speciality Day. AAOS, Atlanta, Georgia, 25 Feb 1996
2. Berger RA (1997) A technique for arthroscopic evaluation of the first carpometacarpal joint. J Hand Surg Am 22(6):1077–1080
3. Bonola A, Caroli A, Celli L (1981) La mano. Piccin Padova 1981
4. Badia A (2006) Trapeziometacarpal arthroscopy: a classification and treatment algorithm. Hand Clin 22:153–163
5. Culp RW, Rekant MS (2001) The role of arthroscopy in evaluating and treating trapeziometacarpal disease. Hand Clin 17:315–319, x–xi

6. Luchetti R, Badia A, Orbay J, Berger R, Atzei A (2001) Artroscopia dell'articolazione trapezio-metacarpica. In: *Artroscopia di polso* Ed Mattioli
7. Pederzini L (1999) *Artroscopia di polso*. Ed Springer
8. Weilby A (1988) Tendon interposition arthroplasty of the first carpometacarpal joint. J Hand Surg Br 13:421
9. Brunelli G, Monini L, Brunelli F (1990) Stabilization de l'articulation trapezo-métacarpien dans les instabilitès et les rhizarthrose débutantes. In: Saffar P (ed) La rhizarthrose. Expansion Scientifique Francaise, Paris, pp 88–92

Surgical Approaches and Techniques

7

Nowadays, in literature, there isn't an evidence of a gold standard treatment in thumb osteoarthritis. In the last decade, a variety of surgical techniques have been described to obtain pain relief, strength, mobility and stability restoration: arthrodesis, trapezial excision, trapezial excision and ligament reconstruction with tendon interposition or without tendon interposition, silicone arthroplasty, Dacron interposition, and total joint implant arthroplasty.

The primary restraints of the trapeziometacarpal joint are anterior oblique ligament and intermetacarpal ligament; to avoid dorsal subluxation, even the beak ligament (palmar oblique) has a fundamental role in joint stability.

Gervis in 1949 proposed the excision of the trapezium; he referred about good results in pain relief and daily function, but this kind of surgery resulted in thumb weakness and instability because of the shortening and subluxation of first metacarpal bone [1].

To avoid this complication, Froimson, in 1970, described the use of rolled-up tendon to fill up the empty space between the first metacarpal bone and trapezium; this procedure can manage shortening but not instability of the thumb [2]. Several authors used silicon implants to restore joint function and to eliminate shortening, but silicone implants resulted in many important complications, implant failure and subluxation, synovitis and bone erosion [3].

Pellegrini e Burton decided to perform partial or total trapeziectomy and to perform a ligament reconstruction using tendon interposition to prevent first metacarpal instability; a radial split of the flexor carpi radialis (FCR) is passed from its distal insertion to the base of first metacarpal bone to stabilize the thumb. In 1995 in order to simplify the technique, they suggested to execute a total trapeziectomy and to use the entire width of FCR tendon [4].

Many authors described different evolutions of this technique; in 1993 Illaramendi and De Carlo suggested to use extensor radialis carpus longus (ERCL) to perform the intermetacarpal ligament reconstruction. Surgery is performed under regional anaesthesia, patient is supine, a pneumatic tourniquet is used on the arm, and a

S. Odella, *Trapeziometacarpal Joint Osteoarthritis*,
https://doi.org/10.1007/978-3-319-44336-2_7

5–6-cm-long incision from the base of second metacarpal to the tip of the radial styloid is performed in order to approach the TMC joint. The abductor pollicis longus, extensor pollicis brevis and extensor pollicis longus tendon are identified; the sensory branches of radialis nerve are retracted and protected. The radial artery is identified in its snuffbox close to the trapezium, if a branch for the capsule of the TMC joint is present, is ligated and is divided. The radial artery is protected. The articular capsule is identified, and a flap is created and carefully dissected from the underlying trapezium preserving the capsule attachment to the base of the first metacarpal. The trapezium is completely excised taking a particular care to remove ulnar osteophyte, protecting FCR tendon; a 5-cm-long distally based radial strip of ECRL tendon is taken between the retinaculum distal border and the second metacarpal. A 4-mm tunnel is drilled at the base of the first metacarpal, and the free end of ERCL is passed under the radial artery and through the metacarpal tunnel from proximal to distal, and the first metacarpal is tight to the second. Thumb stability is tested, the tendon strip is sutured to the distal insertion of the ERCL at the base of the second metacarpal, the capsule is sutured, the thumb is fixed in opposition, and a K-wire is passed through the two metacarpals to protect the ligament reconstruction. The immobilization is recommended at night 6 weeks in a cast; after this the patient will use a night splint for 2 more weeks [5].

The use of FCR tendon for basal joint reconstruction has been associated with weakness in wrist flexion and torsion; Thompson suggested to use the abductor pollicis longus (APL) instead of FCR tendon to recreate the intermetacarpal ligament [6, 7]. Brunelli thought that the use of APL as a sling between the thumb and the index metacarpals converted it in a stabilizing force, avoiding any functional consequence [8].

Kochevar reviewed the long-term results of this technique, a 2-cm-long incision is performed over the dorsal region of the thumb, the first extensor compartment is accessed, and the sheath of the APL and extensor pollicis brevis tendon is split after the trapezium is excised; a 2-cm-long incision is made over the APL at the junction of the middle and the distal third of the forearm; one leash of the APL tendon is identified and divided at the musculotendinous junction; the APL flap is slid by a tendon passer from proximal to distal; a tunnel is drilled at the base of the first metacarpal from the dorsal to volar, and another tunnel is drilled at the base of the second metacarpal from the radio volar to ulnodorsal; the APL flap is passed from the dorsal to volar in the thumb metacarpal, and from volar to dorsal in the second metacarpal tunnel, the graft is passed back inside the wrist, above the extensor carpi radialis longus (ECRL) and volar to the FCR, extensor pollicis longus (EPL) and extensor pollicis brevis (EPB) tendon. The graft is sutured to the periosteum at the base of the first metacarpal under the EPB. A suture is placed even at the crossover point between APL and FCR tendon; to maintain the carpometacarpal joint space, a K-wire is inserted 1 cm distally the base of the metacarpal thumb. A cast is positioned for 8 weeks after surgery [9].

Soejima performed the same technique but applied a splint just for 2 weeks after surgery, and then range-of-motion and grip-strengthening exercises were initiated [10].

Thompson first described this suspensionplasty procedure using the APL tendon to maintain thumb position after trapeziectomy; this procedure allows to minimize proximal and dorsal migration more than simple LRTI arthroplasty; more advantages of this procedure consist in an easier execution of this technique, the APL tendon is removed as a deforming force, and the flexor carpi radialis tendon is preserved as a stabilizer of the wrist.

Belcher and Nicholl reported comparative results of trapeziectomy with and without LRTI performed using APL tendon as a sling and concluded that the addition of a ligament reconstruction did not confer any additional benefit [11].

Some authors have found no correlation between the height of the arthroplasty space and the overall degree of satisfaction in pain relief or improvement in the thumb function and strength [11, 12].

The ideal arthroplasty should reduce or eliminate pain and restore motion and strength; the ligament reconstruction with tendon interposition (LRTI) has similar functional results even if it's performed without tendon interposition or with trapeziectomy alone augmented by a short-term K-wire fixation. The importance of maintaining thumb height and stability of reconstruction remains to have controversial questions; the comparison between LRTI and implant arthroplasty demonstrates more accurately, resembled in normal joint in case of LRTI, implant arthroplasty which resulted in kinematics comparable to other total joints, characterized by a ball and socket axis of rotation with a higher rate of wear and loosening.

Luria and Trumble evaluated the difference in stability achieved after TI, LR and their combination versus the implant arthroplasty in a cadaver model, the implant is in silicon, and it's stabilized using FCR. Thumb pinch is simulated by loading of tendons extensor pollicis longus (EPL), adductor pollicis (ADD), abductor pollicis brevis (APB) and flexor pollicis brevis (FPB), flexor pollicis longus (FPL) and abductor pollicis longus (APL). Authors observed that the implant filled the space remaining after trapeziectomy, restoring its shape and height and keeping the metacarpal base level and trapezial space in its original shape. Neither LR, TIL nor LRTI achieved similar results; there was a significant displacement of the first metacarpal. The ulnar dislocation of the thumb after trapeziectomy could be due to the pull of the adductor muscle and to the tightening of FCR after the LRTI procedure; the rotational instability is more important in case of implant than in case of trapeziectomy alone; probably this rotation instability is due to the fixation of the implant performed distally using FCR; proximally the implant is not secured. The significance of the rotation is not clear; it does not cause subluxation of the implant. They didn't find a biomechanical advantage in the addition of the TI or LR. Author found that the ligament reconstruction caused an increase in the metacarpal base angle compared with the other procedures, which became more pronounced after loading; probably the cause is the deforming force of the FCR tendon. There's no biomechanics advantage in performing LRTI, TI and LR instead of simple trapeziectomy; a stable arthroplasty, aligned with the axis of the excised trapezium, will result in improved range of motion and pinch strength [13].

An interesting review in 2011 compared the eight most popular surgical procedures used to treat trapeziometacarpal arthritis: volar ligament reconstruction, metacarpal osteotomy, carpometacarpal arthrodesis, joint replacement, and trapeziectomy; this last procedure can be performed in a separate treatment or in combination with tendon interposition (TI), ligament reconstruction (LR) or ligament reconstruction in association with tendon interposition (LRTI) [14].

Martou published a systematic review up to 2002, concluding that, even if authors suggested the LRTI is the best procedure, most of these studies included too many methodological flaws to warrant such a treatment suggestion; LRTI does not provide any additional benefit when compared with trapeziectomy alone or in association with TI or with CMC arthrodesis [15].

Wajon from Cochrane Collaboration in 2005 concluded that no procedure is superior to another in terms of pain, physical function, patient global assessment, range of motion or strength; patients who had LRTI had more complications, including scar tenderness, tendon adhesion or rupture, sensory charge or complex regional pain syndrome type 1; patients who had simple trapeziectomy had fewer complications than those who had the other common procedure [16]; in 2009 Wajon updated the Cochrane review, and the firm conclusion is that simple trapeziectomy has less complications than LRTI [17].

Vermeulen considered that volar ligament reconstruction, metacarpal osteotomy, CMC arthrodesis, joint replacement procedures and total joint prosthesis are valuable treatment options in specific patient group; Gervis in 1949 introduced the concept of trapeziectomy without suspension arthroplasty or TI; new materials were introduced to perform interposition instead of tendon such as Gore-Tex or Permacol; the rate of complication was major than before. In literature authors preferred the resection arthroplasty which is technically simpler and has equal result at long-term evaluation compared to trapeziectomy combined with tendon interposition or CMC arthrodesis; shortened surgical time decreases costs and tourniquet and anaesthesia exposure for the patient.

The comparison between trapeziectomy with ligament reconstruction and trapeziectomy with ligament reconstruction and tendon interposition demonstrated that performing LRTI gave no additional benefits over CMC arthrodesis or trapeziectomy with or without TI; Taylor found a higher rate of complications and repeat surgery in the arthrodesis group [18].

Garcia-Mas in 2009 compared total and hemi-trapeziectomy combined with LRTI, they concluded that both resulted in good outcome, but total trapeziectomy should be restricted for stage IV OA [19].

Arthrodesis of the CMC thumb joint is still a valid technique to treat osteoarthrosis; literature referred equal results in pain relief as trapeziectomy combined with LRTI [16–18]. The method of fixation of the arthrodesis, K-wire or plate and screws gave the same outcomes in non-union rates, approximately 8%, but the plate and screws group had lower satisfaction rate, and secondary surgery was more common [20]; thumb CMC arthrodesis is indicated not only for young and demanding patient strength but even in old patients with stage II and III OA [18].

The systematic review of the literature reporting results about trapezial Silastic replacement arthroplasties highlighted a high rate of complications, pain relief and good results but are short term; Silastic implants are associated to long-term complications: subluxations, fractures and silicon synovitis [16, 17].

Total joint replacement was developed in 1970; patients who underwent a joint prosthetic substitution instead of trapeziectomy combined with LRTI had better results in pain relief, strength, range of motion, patient comfort and faster convalescence, without an increased complication rate; implant failure was about 2.8% [21]. Total joint prosthesis is a good option in stage II and III OA; immediate stability, strength and motion are realized, but implant loosening can occur; recent improving quality in total prosthesis could have a significant positive effect on outcomes.

Wilson in 1973 described the basal osteotomy in the treatment of TMC joint; an abduction osteotomy of the proximal end of the thumb metacarpal is performed by removing a radial-based bone wedge and closing the defect by abducting the distal fragment. This technique can be adopted in selected patients with early disease I and II stage OA [22]; in the same years, Eaton and Littler described a ligament volar reconstruction to reconstruct the beak ligament of the symptomatic hypermobile first CMC joint without notable arthritis, using the FCR tendon. This is a good technique in case of articular TMC painful laxity [23].

Considering literature results, it's not still possible to identify the optimal surgical procedure, but some considerations are possible: there's still no evidence that trapeziectomy alone or with interposition or any other technique is superior, but if interposition is performed, it is better to use autologous tendon; non-autologous tissue is associated to increased complications; surgeons are still convinced there's a long-term benefit of LRTI compared to simple trapeziectomy, because despite the evidence that trapeziectomy alone is safer, they continue to perform LRTI. CMC arthrodesis is still a good technique, despite 8% of non-union, and repeat surgery patients are overall satisfied; most of the patients affected by non-union didn't complain about pain, and no added surgery was necessary [24]. Silastic implants are not justified even if they provide a good immediate stability, strength and range-of-motion restoration; long-term complications such as a subluxation, fractured implant and silicon synovitis affect clinical results and patient satisfaction.

At this time, no procedure is superior to another in terms of physical function, patient global assessment, range of motion and strength.

7.1 Algorithm of Treatment

There are many different techniques for the treatment of TMC OA; considering that there isn't one superior to the others, we can perform a different one considering age, daily living activity, range of motion, OA stage, subluxation in X-ray, trapezium morphology and bone stock and cartilage erosion [25].

In initial stages of osteoarthritis, in patients younger than 75 years, with any kind of job, good ROM, stage I OA, metacarpal subluxation minus 40% and no cartilage erosion, the favourite treatment could be sinovialectomy and arthroscopic debridement.

7.2 Technique Description

Portals for arthroscopy of the first carpo metacarpal joint are two, they are named according to their relationship with the EPB and APL. The 1R portal is just radial the APL, tendon at the joint line, the 1-U Portal is just ulnar to the EPB at the joint line.

From the 1-R portal it's possible to view the first mtc, the trapezium, the dorso radial ligament, poterior oblique ligament.

From the 1-U portal it's possible to view first mtc, trapezium, deep portion of the anterior oblique ligament, superficial portion of the anterior oblique ligament.

In patient affected by an initial stage of OA, less than 75 years old, and has any kind of job activity, complete ROM and any degree of trapeziometacarpal subluxation, an interesting option could be extension osteotomy.

Surgical technique: the approach is dorsal, through a straight incision over first metacarpal and trapezium; the sensory branch of the radial nerve is identified and protected and radial artery also. The articular capsule is cut, and the articular cartilage surface and the subchondral bone are removed using a osteotome, small saw blades or dentist drills; a small laminar spreader is interposed to achieve lengthening and correction of the adduction, a corticocancellous bone graft from iliac crest can be interposed to create intrinsic stability and abduction, if necessary the remaining space is filled with cancellous bone, and the fixation can be performed using K-wire or plate and dedicated screws. A splint is necessary for 6–8 weeks; an X-ray check is necessary 40 days after surgery.

Results are satisfying, the method is reliable, and the ROM is not markedly restricted; complication can be easily handled [26].

7.3 Surgical Approaches and Techniques: Interposition Implants and TM Joint Fusion

In patients affected by stage II OA, 65–70 years old, non-hard worker, ROM complete, non-trapeziometacarpal subluxation, non-trapezial dysplasia, in presence of a good bone stock, important cartilage erosion, a valid solution could be the pyrocarbon metacarpal hemi-prosthesis.

Surgical technique: The procedure is performed under either general or axillary block anaesthesia, under an upper arm tourniquet. Fluoroscopy is used to visualize bone resection, alignment, broaching and placement of the trial implant and prosthesis. Our standard approach is a longitudinal dorsal incision over the thumb metacarpal base and carpus between the extensor pollicis longus and abductor pollicis longus (APL) tendons. Dissection is extended down through the subcutaneous tissues, and the superficial branches of the radial nerve and the dorsal branch of the radial artery are identified and carefully preserved.

A longitudinal incision is made on the metacarpal base and dorsal capsule overlying the trapezium between the extensor pollicis longus and APL tendons until the scaphotrapezial joint is identified. Medial and lateral capsular flaps are then elevated keeping them as thick as possible. A small arthrotomy is then made in the scaphotrapezial joint and the joint palpated with a Freer elevator to determine any loss of cartilage. The articular surface of the trapezium with the metacarpal base is then inspected to determine the suitability for using a Saddle implant or whether to create a concavity in the trapezium for placement of a PyroHemiSphere or NuGrip implant. Independent of implant choice, a starter awl is used to make a puncture hole just under the dorsal cortex of the midpoint of the base of the metacarpal. The cutting alignment guide is inserted into the medullary cavity of the metacarpal and its position checked on postero-anterior and lateral fluoroscopy. The appropriate cutting guide is then attached, and a small thin oscillating saw is used to make a perpendicular cut through the metacarpal base approximately 3 mm from the articular surface if the Saddle implant is to be used or a 27.5-degree angle cut if the PyroHemiSphere or NuGrip implants are to be used. After placement of the trial implant, this osteotomy may have to be revised to remove slightly more bone from the metacarpal base. The sizing template is used to determine the size of the distal articular surface of the trapezium. The Saddle implant comes in four sizes – 10, 20, 30 and 40 mm – but most of our cases have used the 20-mm implant. Once the size of the implant has been determined, sequential broaching is performed up to the correct size, paying attention to position the broach directly down the centre of the medullary canal just beneath the dorsal cortex. The position of the broach is confirmed on fluoroscopy. If the Saddle implant is to be used, the trial implant is inserted into the metacarpal and allowed to articulate with the trapezium, and the joint is passively ranged through abduction, adduction and flexion to ensure that there is no impingement of the cut edges of the metacarpal base on the trapezium. Fluoroscopy is repeated to confirm proper alignment and articulation. If the PyroHemiSphere or NuGrip implant is to be used, a round or pineapple burr is used to create a socket for the head of the implant in the central area of the trapezium, and fluoroscopy is again used to check positioning.

The trial implant is removed, and capsular reconstruction is begun before placement of the final implant. A 0.035-in. K-wire is used to drill two holes in the dorsal surface of metacarpal approximately 5 mm away from the cut edge. A double-armed 3-0 or 4-0 permanent suture is passed from inside the medullary canal out through each of the two holes and secured in a haemostat. The final implant is then secured into position with a tamp and mallet. The previously placed suture is inserted proximally through each of the medial and lateral capsular flaps and tied with the thumb in extension, thus advancing the flaps distally. If necessary, one of the slips of the APL tendon may be incorporated in this closure to advance the slip more distally, to tighten the capsule and to reinforce the capsular repair. The capsular flaps are approximated completely, and reinforcing sutures are inserted to ensure a secure reconstruction. Position and stability of the final implant is confirmed on fluoroscopy. Once adequate positioning and stability have been confirmed, the tourniquet is deflated and haemostasis achieved. The skin is closed with interrupted 4-0 nylon horizontal mattress sutures. A nonadhesive dressing is placed over the suture line and a plaster of Paris thumb spica splint applied with the thumb in extension and moderate abduction, to allow scar formation to heal the dorsal capsule with the implant in anatomic position and prevent dorsal subluxation.

After surgery, a splint is positioned for 2 weeks including interphalangeal joint; after this period a cast for 4 more weeks is used by the patient; this is crucial for the healing of the dorsal capsule to avoid dorsal subluxation and pain. At 6 weeks, an X-ray is taken to check the position of the implant, and gentle active exercises are started. The patient is instructed not to do any passive flexion of the thumb at the carpometacarpal or metacarpophalangeal joints until after 3 months, when strengthening exercises for pinch and grasp can be started. This procedure prevents shortening and subsidence of the thumb so often seen with trapezial resection or tendon interposition arthroplasty, which eventually results in decreased pinch and grip strength. In addition, failure of this pyrocarbon implant arthroplasty does not preclude salvage with a conventional resection arthroplasty [27].

In case of patients 65–70 years old, non-hard worker, complete ROM, stage III OA, scapho-trapezio-trapezoide joint safe, trapeziometacarpal subluxation minus than 40%, non-trapezial dysplasia and valid bon stock, extended cartilage erosion, preferred surgical treatment is complete implant arthroplasty. In authors' experience the used implant is the SR prosthesis.

7.3.1 Prosthesis Design

The SR TMC prosthesis (Avanta Orthopaedics) consists of two components whose saddle-like articular surfaces are congruent and have slightly greater curvature than the anatomic surfaces to provide increased stability.

The trapezial component is a chrome cobalt alloy with a rounded peg for anchorage within the centre of the trapezial surface. The peg is designed to fit in a hole drilled in the central position of the distal articular surface of the trapezium. The rough undersurface of the proximal component provides for a wider contact area.

The metacarpal (MC) component is made of ultrahigh-molecular-weight polyethylene. The articular surface is displaced palmarly approximately 3 mm relative to the stem to correspond to the anatomic offset of the first MC shaft. The stem is slab-sided to make orientation after insertion easier to judge.

7.3.2 Surgical Technique

Under tourniquet control and adequate anaesthesia, a V-shaped incision with an angle of 90° is made over the TMC joint distal to the snuffbox, with the apex of the incision located at the junction between the dorsal and palmar skin [4]. The branches of the superficial sensory radial nerve are identified and protected. The deep fascia over the anatomic snuffbox is incised, and the radial artery and its vena are mobilized.

The posterior capsule is incised to either side of the trapezium, and the lines are extended distally into the periosteum along either side of the proximal first MC. A transverse incision is made in the periosteum 1.5 cm from the base of the MC. The periosteum and posterior capsule then are reflected proximally as a flap that will be used to effect later closure. The abductor pollicis longus is released from its MC base insertion and tagged with a suture.

A small sagittal saw is used to remove the proximal 3–4 mm of the first MC perpendicular to the longitudinal axis. The first MC is flexed forward to expose the trapezial surface. There is often an ulnar osteophyte that should be removed to ensure that the prosthesis will be oriented appropriately. A trial proximal component is now placed against the trapezium to ensure the correct component size is selected (the size of the components is estimated preoperatively by placing the templates over the X-ray).

The distal surface of the trapezium is then contoured using the corresponding size of the rotatory burr. This burr removes cartilage and a partial thickness of subchondral bone, necessary to obtain a close fit to the underside of the proximal prosthetic component. The drill hole for the prosthetic peg then is made by using the metal template with the centring hole by inserting it into the joint. The drill bit is aligned perpendicular to the trapezial surface and drilled to the stop on the drill shank. The trial proximal component then is seated onto the trapezium, and the fit and stability are assessed carefully. The long axis of the component should form an 80° angle with the plane through the second and third MC and a 40° angle perpendicular to the second MC in the plane between the first and second MC.

The trapezial trial is removed, and the intramedullary cavity of the first MC is then prepared with the custom broaches. The distal trial component is inserted, being careful to orient the straighter posterior surface facing the surgeon. The proximal aspects of the device should extend about 3 mm above the cutting surface of the MC base.

Then both trial components are inserted again (the proximal one first). Thumb motion is assessed, and position and orientation are checked. When satisfied with the position, stability and motion, the trial components are removed, and the joint space is lavaged. The raw bony surfaces are dried, and methyl methacrylate bone cement is injected. The permanent components then are inserted, being careful to obtain correct orientation. Excess cement must be removed.

The abductor pollicis longus tendon then is reinserted with 3.0 non-absorbable sutures through holes in the bone and sutured to the adjacent periosteum when possible. The posterior capsule is closed by suturing the osteoperiosteal flap securely around its edges with non-absorbable sutures. The tourniquet is released, and bleeding is controlled before completing skin closure.

Finally, a compressive bandage and an immobilizing forearm splint holding the thumb in a position of natural opposition to the index finger tip is applied. Ten days later the splint is replaced by an orthosis, and rehabilitation is started. After 6 weeks, the orthosis is removed permanently [28].

Total joint implant arthroplasty gives stability, strength and mobility even if this procedure is associated to a variable percentage of failure, 10% in cemented prosthesis and 46% in noncemented prosthesis [29, 30]. There are different designs of TMC arthroplasty, but most of them are variations on the constrained ball-and-socket concept. As mentioned by Linscheid, constrained or semi-constrained designs transmit more stress to the stem-bone interface (owing to the small contact area) than a surface replacement arthroplasty. On the other hand, the minimal joint resection that surface replacement arthroplasty requires leaves a wider cortical and trabecular contact surface area for distribution of the joint compressive loads [31]. The SR prosthesis has benefits from an unconstrained design and a minimal resection to minimize failure rates, and the anatomical design should restore the normal kinematics; best results are obtained in older patients probably because of lower demand activity. Literature referred a percentage of good and excellent results around 40%; this is not enough to suggest this procedure as an adequate surgical option treatment for thumb carpometacarpal OA, but this technique can be used just in selected patients.

A different kind of complete prosthesis is the constrained ball-and-socket implant. Historically, the de la Caffiniere implant was the most widely used and most extensively studied implant, but it is no longer commercially available. The Braun prosthesis is now used; the concept is similar, and it can be implanted just in selected patients, who are old and have low-demanding daily life [32].

Surgical approach for thumb basal joint arthroplasty consists of a 3- to 4-cm longitudinal lazy S incision performed over the dorsum at the base of the thumb. This curvilinear incision is a smaller incision that permits better side-to-side retraction. It is also less apparent than simple straight lines. Branches of the superficial sensory radial nerve are identified and protected. Further dissection is carried between the extensor pollicis longus and extensor pollicis brevis tendons protecting the dorsal branch of the radial artery. The dorsal capsule of the trapeziometacarpal joint is opened longitudinally. A transverse incision of about 1.5 cm is made in the periosteum at the base of the metacarpal, also elevating the insertion of the abductor pollicis brevis. The periosteum and the dorsal capsule are reflected proximally as a single flap so that it can be repaired later. A small sagittal saw is used to remove the proximal 8- to 10-mm base of the metacarpal. This manoeuvre facilitates complete release of the joint capsule and the adductor pollicis from the metacarpal shaft. This step allows abduction of the thumb metacarpal away from the palm to improve hand function. At this point, longitudinal traction and flexion are applied to better expose the trapezial surface. A rongeur is used to remove the marginal osteophytes. A high-speed burr or the rasp in the tray is used to create a deep channel within the trapezium or can be used where the polyethylene cup is to be cemented. For the thumb metacarpal, two broaches of different sizes are available for preparing the metacarpal canal and allowing the component to have a generous cement mantle. Both sides of the joint are prepared for implant placement by irrigating them with antibiotic solution and drying the cancellous bony surfaces with gauze. The cup is cemented in the trapezium. Once the cup has been inserted and the cement cured, a second batch of cement is placed in the metacarpal, and the metacarpal component is inserted. As this stem is collarless, adequate neck length must be maintained after insertion so that dislocation does not occur. Dislocation can occur when the stem neck impinges on the edge of the trapezium because of inadequate placement. After proper hardening of this component, the stem is pressed into place in the cup, and stability and circumferential motion are assessed with no impingement on the implant. Any excess cement is excised. With experience, the surgeon can cement both sides of the joint in one stage, considerably shortening operative time. The periosteum-capsule flap is closed with absorbable suture, and meticulous haemostasis is achieved. Intraoperative fluoroscopy is used to check proper alignment and placement of the prosthesis. I typically close the skin with 4-0 Vicryl Rapide (Ethicon, Inc., Somerville, NJ) and apply a well-padded short-arm thumb spica splint with the thumb in opposition (worn for 2 weeks). At this time, rehabilitation is started, and an Orthoplast thumb-based spica splint is indicated for further protection during certain activities. Patients rapidly regain thumb-to-base-of-small-finger opposition with a gentle, active-assisted range-of-motion protocol.

In the event that a volar capsulodesis is needed, a Bruner-type incision is made over the palmar aspect of the metacarpophalangeal joint. The flexor pollicis longus tendon is identified and reflected and the A1 pulley released. Then a U-shaped incision is made on the volar plate to create a distally based flap. The metacarpophalangeal joint is then held in 10° of flexion, and the proximal end of the volar plate is reattached more proximally to the metacarpal neck with a suture anchor with enough tension to maintain the desired degree of flexion. In these cases, a short-arm thumb spica cast up to the interphalangeal joint is used for 1 month.

In selected patients, this technique can give good results in strength, ROM and pain relief and is not suggested in young patients.

In patients that are affected by OA stage II or III, concentric, non-hard worker in presence of a complete ROM and have a good bone stock, the correct option could be a hemi-trapeziectomy with synthetic or biological implant.

Pyrocarbon is a ceramic material obtained from a graphite substrate heated to 1400° in a special oven and placed into a condition of weightlessness by injecting gas under pressure. Carbon and hydrogen bonds of a hydrocarbon gas are broken at the temperature of about 1400°. The union of carbon atoms results in a thick layer on the graphite substrate with a random pattern.

In addition to its properties which are useful for surgical purposes, it has significant advantages for other uses:

It has an exceptional resistance to wear. Pyrocarbon is virtually resistant to damage from its rubbing against itself due to its very low coefficient of friction; this material allows full control of the material's porosity; it has a total chemical inertness which confers complete resistance to corrosion.

The real growth of pyrocarbon use in orthopaedics began in the 1980s. It was focused on use in the upper extremities. Experience of more than 10 years of clinical follow-up has demonstrated the absence of particles resulting from wear [33].

The achievements of pyrocarbon are amazing compared to carbon fibres and other materials of this type that were unsuccessfully used in the past.

Its main characteristics make it an exceptional material that is particularly suited for orthopaedic applications:

- Excellent biocompatibility
- Very low coefficient of friction, especially against bone and cartilage, preventing wear and inflammation
- Modulus of elasticity similar to bone allowing excellent transmission of bone and implant stresses and thereby reducing the patient's pain

In fact, the elastic modulus of pyrocarbon is similar to cortical bone resulting in biomechanical compatibility with bone. Unlike surgical grade metals, pyrocarbon transfers load from implant to bone more effectively, thus reducing stress shielding and potential bone resorption.

The devices projected for the thumb OA are two: PyroDisc and Pyrocardan.

The PyroDisk™ CMC implant is a biarticular convex disc made of pyrocarbon, designed to resurface the thumb carpometacarpal (CMC) joint damaged by arthritis. The implant and CMC joint are stabilized by the flexor carpi radialis tendon, transferred and passed through the trapezium, through the implant and into the first metacarpal (Fig. 7.1).

7.3.3 Surgical Technique

7.3.3.1 Initial Incision and Capsular Exposure

A longitudinal incision is made along the radial base of the first metacarpal passing ulnarward at the wrist flexion crease (Fig. 7.2).

At this time it is necessary to identify, retract and protect the cutaneous branches of the radial nerve and the radial artery. A longitudinal incision of the capsule is made over the dorsum of the metacarpal from 2 cm distal to the CMC joint to the level of the trapezium. With sharp dissection, the CMC joint is identified and entered transversely to remove synovium present (Fig. 7.3).

7.3.3.2 Metacarpal and Trapezial Resections

Use Ragnell retractors to expose the base of the metacarpal. An oscillating saw is used to remove 2–3 mm of bone from the metacarpal base. The trapezial saddle is

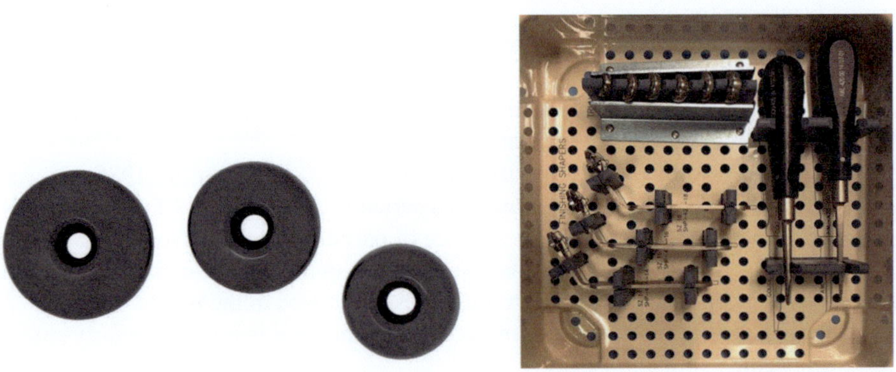

Fig. 7.1 The PyroDisk™ CMC implant and surgical instruments

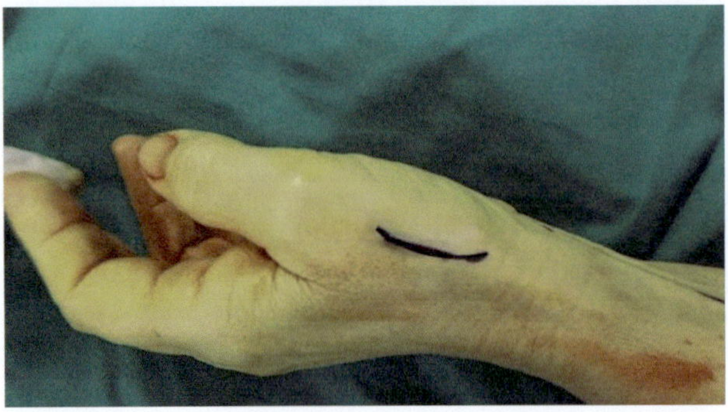

Fig. 7.2 Longitudinal cutaneous incision on the CMC joint, isolation of the sensitive branches of the radial nerve and artery, capsulotomy

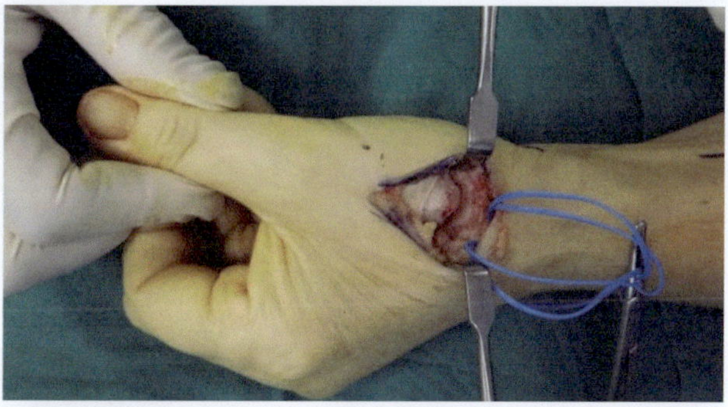

Fig. 7.3 The TMC joint is identified, and the inflammatory synovium is removed

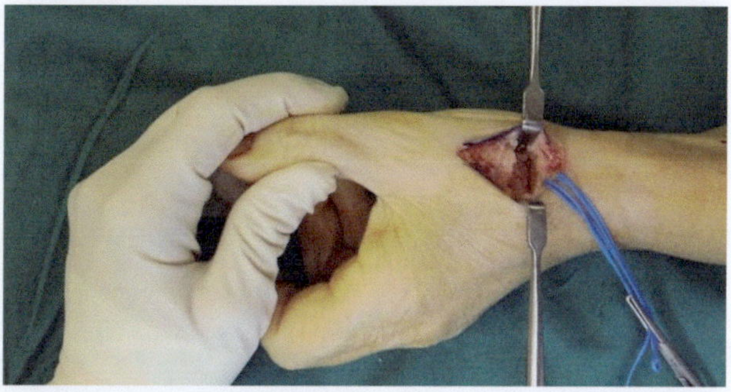

Fig. 7.4 Partial trapeziectomy is performed using oscillating saw; the cartilage layer, subchondral bone and osteophytes are removed. An oscillating saw is used to remove 2–3 mm of bone from the metacarpal base. Trapezium and the base of the first metacarpal bone must be parallel

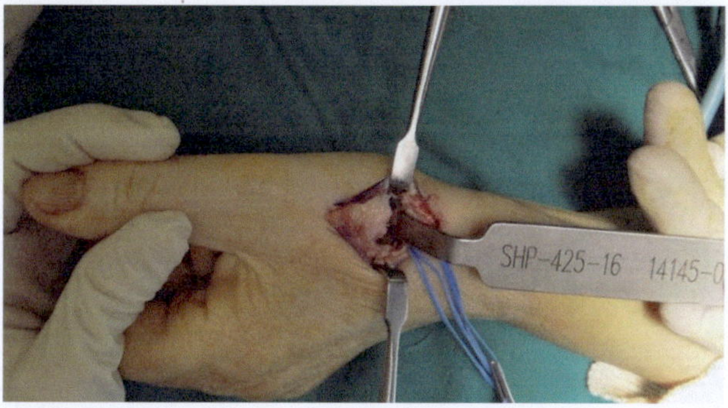

Fig. 7.5 The first metacarpal base and the trapezium are shaped using a dedicated broach

then flattened with the oscillating saw preserving as much trapezial height as possible, while removing the medial and lateral horns for a smooth surface that is parallel to the metacarpal cut (Fig. 7.4).

It often takes a small rongeur to thoroughly remove the fragments from the trapezial cut, as well as any medial or lateral osteophytes that may be present.

7.3.3.3 Metacarpal and Trapezial Broaching

The Ascension broach is used to create a concave surface at the base of the metacarpal and distal surface of the trapezium. Centre the broach over the recessed surface of the trapezium and the metacarpal. Compress the joint while rotating the broach back and forth to create the shallow recesses. Trapezial bone is quite hard and often requires additional gentle burring with a small round burr to achieve the proper configuration (Fig. 7.5).

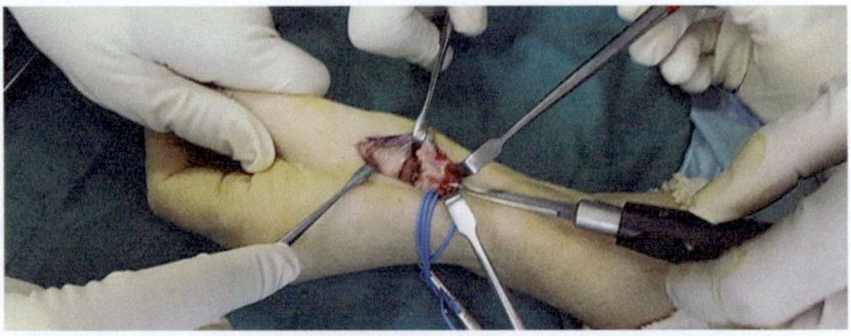

Fig. 7.6 Trapezial tunnel preparation

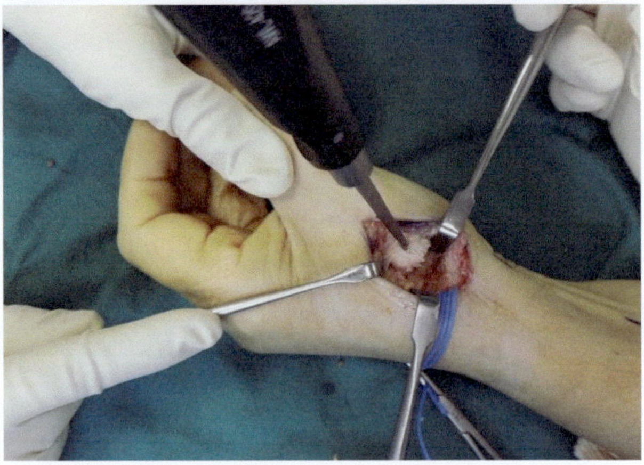

Fig. 7.7 First metacarpal base tunnel preparation

7.3.3.4 Trapezial Preparation

Using the starter awl, a hole is created through the centre of the trapezium. This is accomplished by creating a small pilot hole in the centre of the proximal radial surface of the trapezium and then passing the tip of the awl into the resected joint at the distal surface of the trapezium. The hole diameter should be approximately 3.5 mm. A power drill can be used, but there is a risk of trapezial fracture (Fig. 7.6).

7.3.3.5 Metacarpal Preparation

The starter awl is used to open up a tunnel in the medullary canal of the metacarpal. This tunnel is connected to a second hole created through the dorsal cortex of the metacarpal – approximately 12 mm distal to the resection at the base of the metacarpal. A hand gouge is used to gently enlarge these holes to prevent fraying of the tendon during passage (Fig. 7.7).

7.3.3.6 Trial Reduction

Insert the trial implant size estimated preoperatively using the X-ray templates, and reduce the joint. Lightly compress the joint, and verify that the appropriate size has been selected. Care is taken to select a prosthesis that closely matches but does not exceed the diameter of the base of the metacarpal. Remove the implant trial (Fig. 7.8a–d).

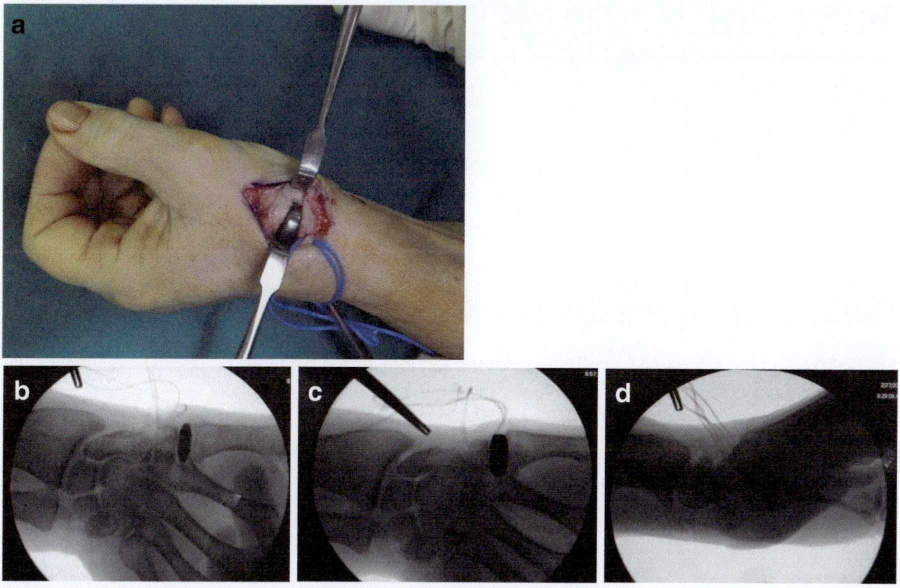

Fig. 7.8 (**a**) The trial is inserted; (**b–d**) X-ray control

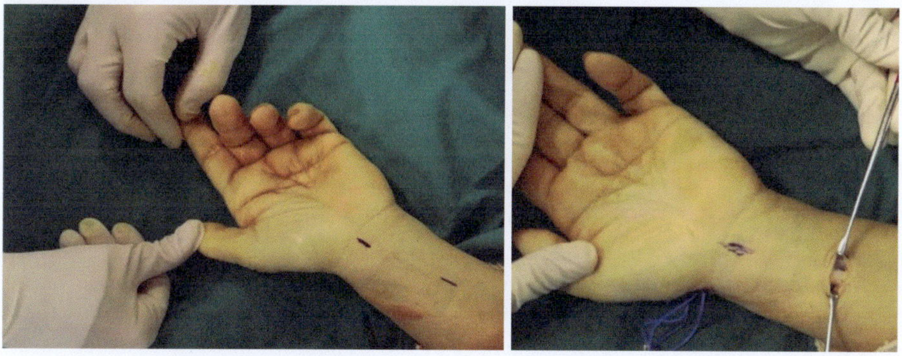

Fig. 7.9 The ulnar side of FCR is harvested

7.3.3.7 Harvesting the Tendon

Two small transverse incisions in the forearm permit harvesting of the radial half of the flexor carpi radialis tendon (Fig. 7.9).

By wrist positioning in various degrees of flexion, a great part of the tendon can be visualized as the sheath of the tendon is released and the tendon is stripped either through gentle traction or scissor dissection to the base of the thenar muscles. The thickness of the harvested tendon should allow clearance through the 3.5-mm hole in the centre of the PyroDisk® implant. The tendon is passed stepwise from the proximal incision to the middle incision and then similarly to the area at the tuberosity of the scaphoid. With the tendon freed to this level, it is then passed gently

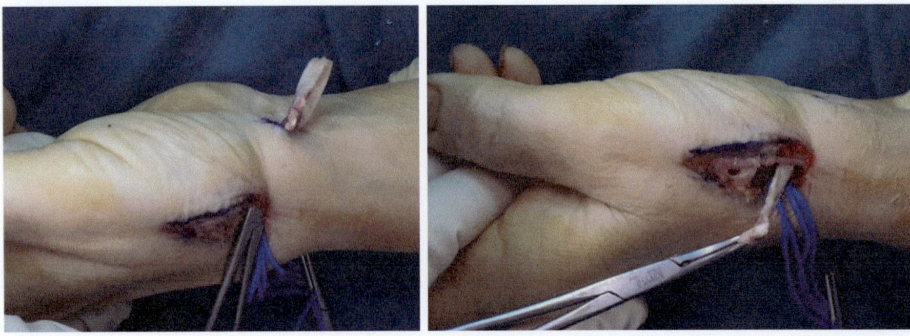

Fig. 7.10 The tendon passed gently beneath the tendons of the first compartment to the rim of the proximal aspect of the trapezium where the previous hole has been created

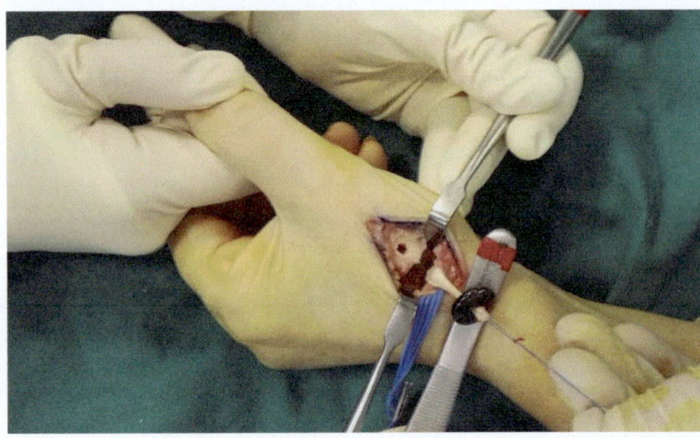

Fig. 7.11 FCR is passed through trapezium tunnel PyroDisc and first metacarpal tunnel

beneath the tendons of the first compartment to the rim of the proximal aspect of the trapezium where the previous hole has been created (Fig. 7.10).

7.3.3.8 Passing the Tendon Graft

The tendon graft is then passed through the hole in the trapezium from the proximal aspect out through the distal aspect of the trapezium into the resected joint. The properly selected Ascension® PyroDisk® implant is opened. The tendon is placed through the hole in the properly selected Ascension® PyroDisk® implant, then into the first metacarpal to exit through the dorsal hole in the first metacarpal (Fig. 7.11).

7.3.3.9 Final Close

With the tendon pulled snugly, the first metacarpal is held in radial and palmar abduction, while a firm capsular closure is achieved with 4-0 PDS or appropriate absorbable suture. The end of the tendon is used for capsular reinforcement, and after three or four appropriate sutures, the end of the tendon can then be passed back beneath the muscles of the first compartment to be secured to the remaining flexor carpi radialis, just proximal to the tuberosity of the scaphoid (Fig 7.12).

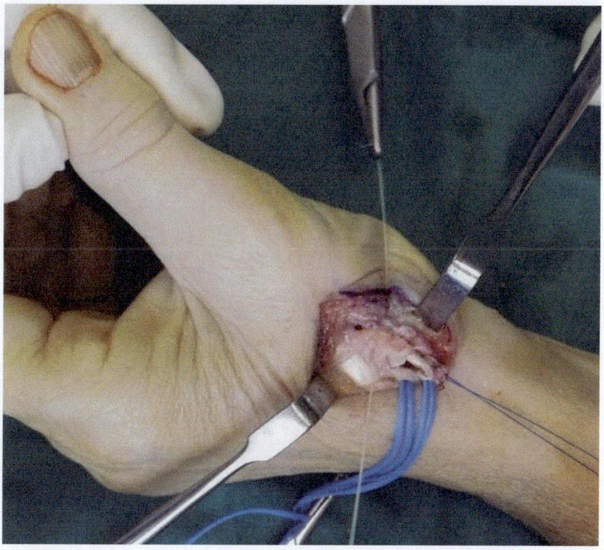

Fig. 7.12 With the tendon pulled snugly, the first metacarpal is held in radial and palmar abduction, while a firm capsular closure is achieved

All incisions are irrigated and closed with 5-0 nylon. A well-padded sterile dressing is applied with a loose fibreglass case maintaining the wrist in neutral or 20° of extension and the thumb metacarpal in comfortable palmar and radial abduction. A final X-ray is then performed.

Postoperative treatment considers a splint of immobilization for 4 weeks, and then after an X-ray check, the patient can start exercises of hand mobilizations, avoiding charges for 1 more month (Fig. 7.13).

The patient must be informed about the durability of the pain that could be even 6 months from surgery; this procedure permits to obtain good results in strength, ROM, thumb length and pain relief, a low rate of complications and in particularly low rate of revision surgery. Even though Iogoe et al. [34] recently reported better results in patients treated by trapeziectomy than in ones treated by interposition implant, we believe that the PyroDisk is a good solution in selected patients (Eaton stages I–III disease without subluxation).

Pyrocardan is a free resurfacing implant made of pyrocarbon for the trapeziometacarpal joint.

Its compact size (thickness of 1 mm) allows for a very simple and minimally invasive surgical procedure.

The Pyrocardan®'s very specific design (two orthogonal and concave surfaces) corresponds to the main curvature of the metacarpal on one hand and of the trapezium on the other, thereby reproducing the anatomical trapeziometacarpal joint and allowing the stability of the implant [1].

The Pyrocardan® is a choice solution for treating painful early-stage TMC arthritis; the advantages of this treatment are the minimally invasive technique, in fact it's possible to spare ligament insertion and preserve bone stock (minimal resection and articulation centre sparing); the interposition is very thin (1 mm in the middle of the implant);

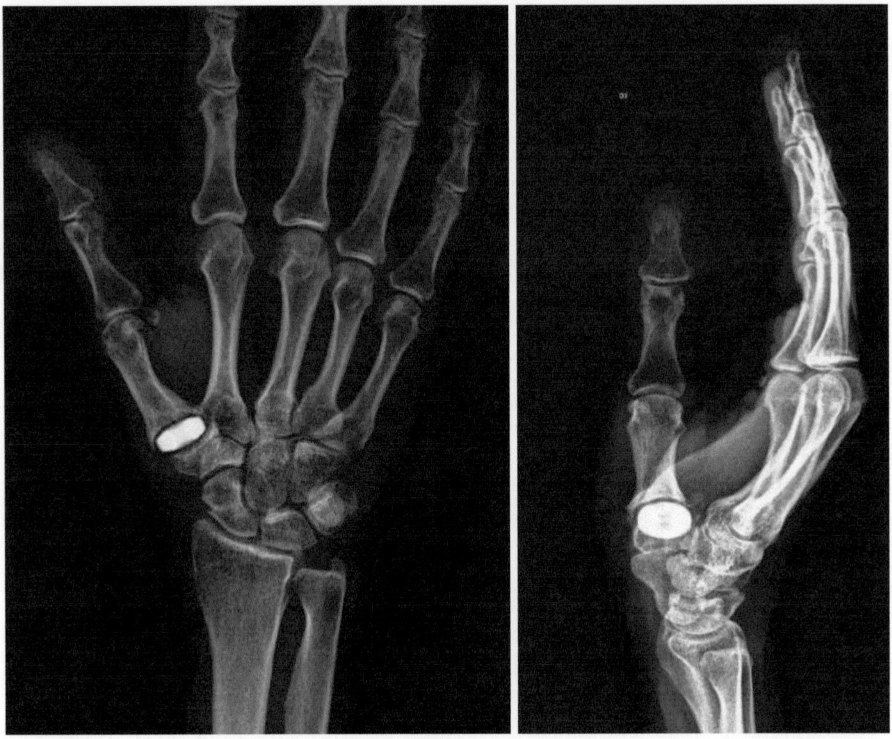

Fig. 7.13 One-month postoperative follow-up X-ray. The implant is well positioned; no bone reabsorption is highlighted

the implant is anatomical, free and stable; it allows to adapt its position to dynamic shearing of forces, having movements similar to physiological TMC double saddle. In case of failure, it's possible to perform a traditional technique. The Pyrocardan (Tornier SAS, Etablissement Bioprofile, France) is a rectangular-shaped implant made from two tubular concavities opposed perpendicularly to one another (Fig. 7.14). In its centre the implant is 1-mm thick. The thickness of the edge of the implant depends on its size. Six sizes are available for the use in the TM joint. They are defined by the length of the implant measured in millimetres and ranking from 14 (XS) to 18 (XXL). The implant is positioned in the TM joint so that its length is in the lateromedial axis of the joint line and its anteroposterior concavity is opposed to the trapezial joint surface.

Surgical technique: The skin incision is dorsal and slightly distal to the posterior part of the first metacarpal; the tendon of the extensor pollicis longus is protected to the medial side of the incision and the tendon of the extensor pollicis brevis to the lateral side to expose the base of first metacarpal. A rectangular capsulo-periosteal flap is cut out from the base of the metacarpal at an average of 10 mm distal to the joint and between the insertion of the abductor pollicis longus laterally and a line prolonging the ulnar edge of the metacarpal. The capsulo-periosteal flap remains attached proximally and is folded over to expose the joint line. Intra-articular bony resections are done with a thin oscillating saw.

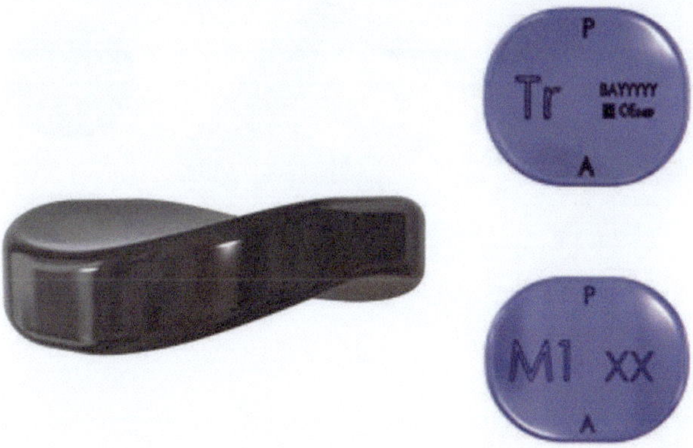

Fig. 7.14 Pyrocardan implant and trial: rectangular-shaped implant made from two tubular concavities opposed perpendicularly to one another

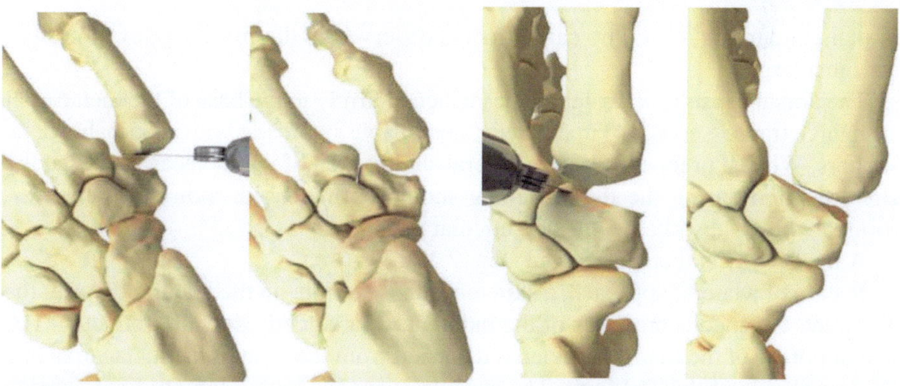

Fig. 7.15 Tornier Technique. The dorsal and palmar edges of the metacarpal are sawed off to smooth its dorso-palmar concavity; on the trapezium the medial horn, which is often prolonged by an osteophyte, is removed

The dorsal and palmar edges of the metacarpal are sawed off to smooth its dorso-palmar concavity. On the trapezium the medial horn, which is often prolonged by an osteophyte, is removed. Its lateral horn is less protruding and can be removed with a saw, a rongeur or a burr. When the joint line is very oblique, the medial horn is resected even more to obtain a horizontal joint line perpendicular to the metacarpal axis and the first column (Fig. 7.15a, b).

It's crucial that bone resections are parallel to the radial axis.

Joint synovectomy is done with a thin rongeur. Special care is taken to free the recess palmar of the trapezium and to resect the osteophyte that often forms there. An ovoid burr is used to smooth the bone cuts. The metacarpal side is roughly shaped into a sphere. The trapezial side is shaped into a straight medio-lateral cut with an anteroposterior convexity. The final implant size is chosen, among a set of trial implants, so that the trapezium is totally covered (Fig. 7.16). Control fluoroscopy is used to check the proper size and positioning of the

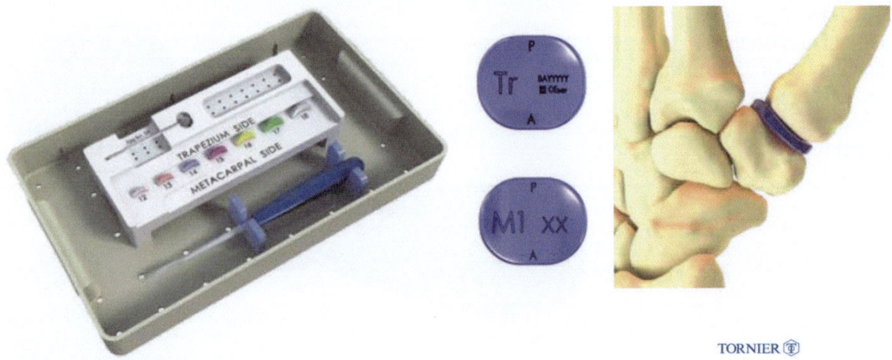

Fig. 7.16 A set of trial implants, the correct size is the one that covers the trapezium surface

implant and to make sure no cam effect is observed in the full range of motion of the metacarpal.

The dorsal capsulo-periosteal flap is fastened firmly to the base of the metacarpal with three transosseous, 3/0 in diameter, absorbable sutures or with absorbable bone anchors. When a preoperative dorsolateral subluxation of the metacarpal exists, the stress applied during the flap fastening should be increased. Skin closure is performed with an absorbable 4/0 subcuticular suture.

A final X-ray is then performed (Fig. 7.17).

In case of a lateral approach, a skin incision is straight on the lateral border of the TM joint. Cutaneous branches of the radial nerve are gently dorsally retracted. The lateral border of the thenar muscles is detached from the base of the metacarpal and the lateral side of the TM joint. The capsule is opened with a longitudinal incision palmarly to the APL tendon.

Bone resections are then performed from lateral to medial on the trapezial and metacarpal saddles. The further joint preparation and placement of the trial implant and the final implant are similar to the dorsal approach procedure. For closure, the two edges of the capsule are reattached and the thenar muscles replaced over it and their fascia reattached.

A thick dressing ensures immediate postoperative immobilization and is replaced the following day by a removable thermoplastic splint. The patient is advised to wear the splint at all times during 15 days until the dressing is removed. Reeducation exercises of the first column are done by the patient starting from the 15th day on, according to a written protocol given to the patient. After the 15th day, the splint should be worn if needed only at night or during manual activities during the day until the 4th week.

Bellemere reported good results in pain relief, strength, ROM and patient satisfaction; he considered this implant promising, and he thinks this is a good option in working patients in stage I or II of OA [3, 35].

The execution of the surgical technique must be very precise; in some cases the implant was painful even if at the X-ray the implant was correct; it's preferable that

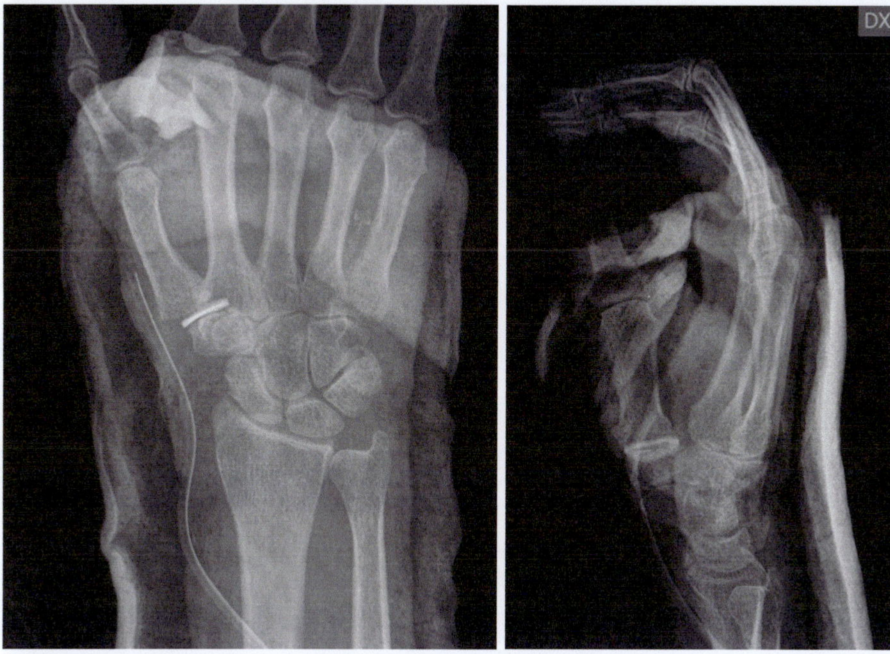

Fig. 7.17 Post-surgery X-ray, the hand is protected in a cast

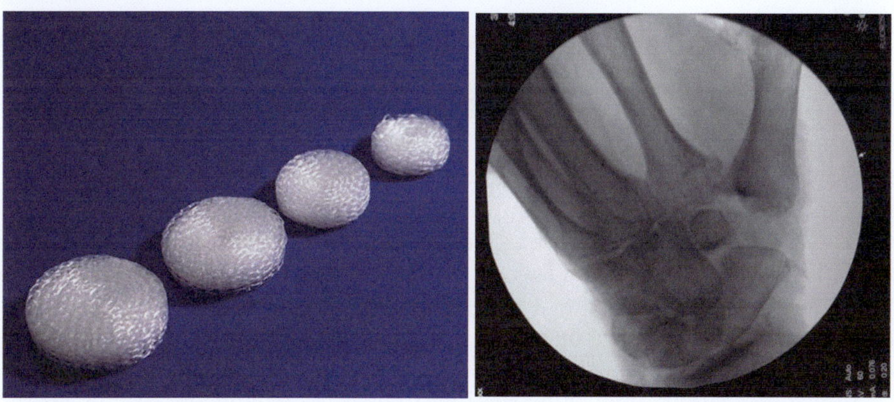

Fig. 7.18 RegJoint™ and intraoperative X-ray view after implant, the implant is not visible at X-ray

the Pyrocardan is oversized; in fact if the implant is too small, a trapezial collapse can occur [36, 37].

Another new material is the one that constitute RegJoint. RegJoint™ is produced from bioabsorbable poly-96L/4D-lactide copolymer fibre (Fig. 7.18). It is a porous, disc-like implant. Due to bioabsorbable material, there is no risk of implant

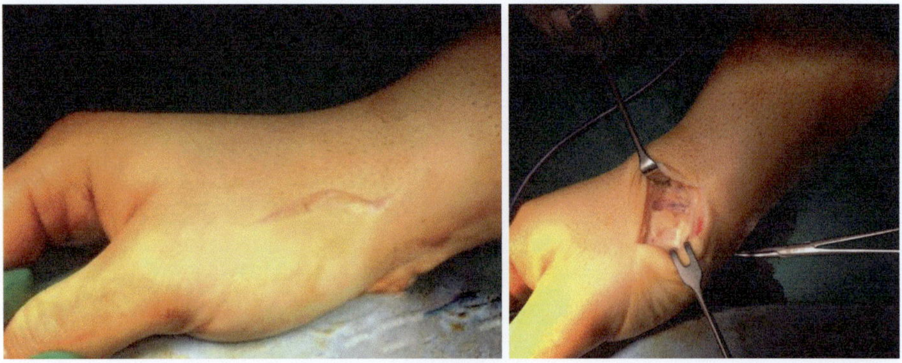

Fig. 7.19 Dorsal incision is performed preserving radial artery

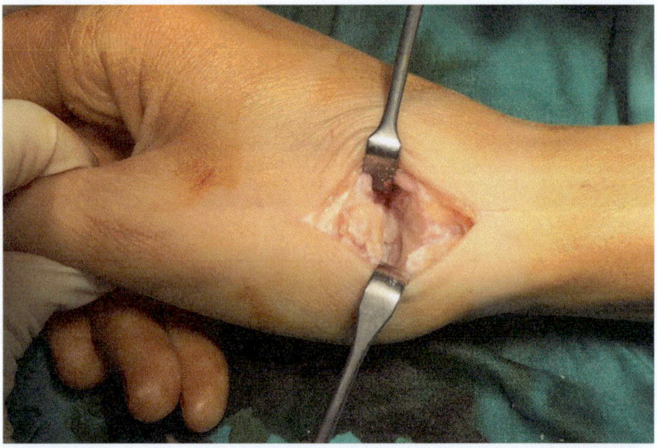

Fig. 7.20 The first metacarpal base is removed using an oscillating saw; the trapezium cartilage surface is removed as the medial osteophyte when it's necessary

breakage and no need for implant removal. However, the restoration of the structure and function are maintained after implant resorption.

RegJoint™ loses its initial strength during 15–24 weeks in vivo, with complete strength loss and resorption on average within 2–3 years, depending on the patient variables. RegJoint™ provides temporary support and guidance for soft tissue ingrowth. It allows a gradual optimized replacement of the implant with fibrous tissue providing a flexible and durable pseudo joint.

Surgical technique: Implanting RegJoint™ does not require any specific instrumentation. All used instruments need to be appropriately cleaned and sterilized before use. All sutures and other materials need to be sterile.

RegJoint™ is sterilized by gamma irradiation and is supplied sterile and ready for use. RegJoint™ shall not be resterilized by any method.

Dorsoradial longitudinal incision preserves branches of superficial radial nerve and the deep branch of the radial artery. The first carpometacarpal (CMC) joint is identified and the capsule released and opened dorsoradially (Fig. 7.19).

The first metacarpal is released carefully proximally to correct the prevailing adduction contracture. The resection of the proximal part of the first metacarpal is done by using an oscillating saw. The resection line of the proximal part of the first metacarpal is perpendicular with respect to the metacarpal. The resection of the cartilage surface of the trapezium is performed using a curette or an oscillating saw (Fig. 7.20).

Other options are partial or complete trapezium resections without metacarpal resection. The extension of the resection is proportional to the joint laxity. Performing synovectomy and revising osteophytes are necessary. RegJoint™ sizers can be used to evaluate the correct size of the implant. Ideal size completely covers the bone end at the fluoroscopic intraoperative control (Fig 7.21).

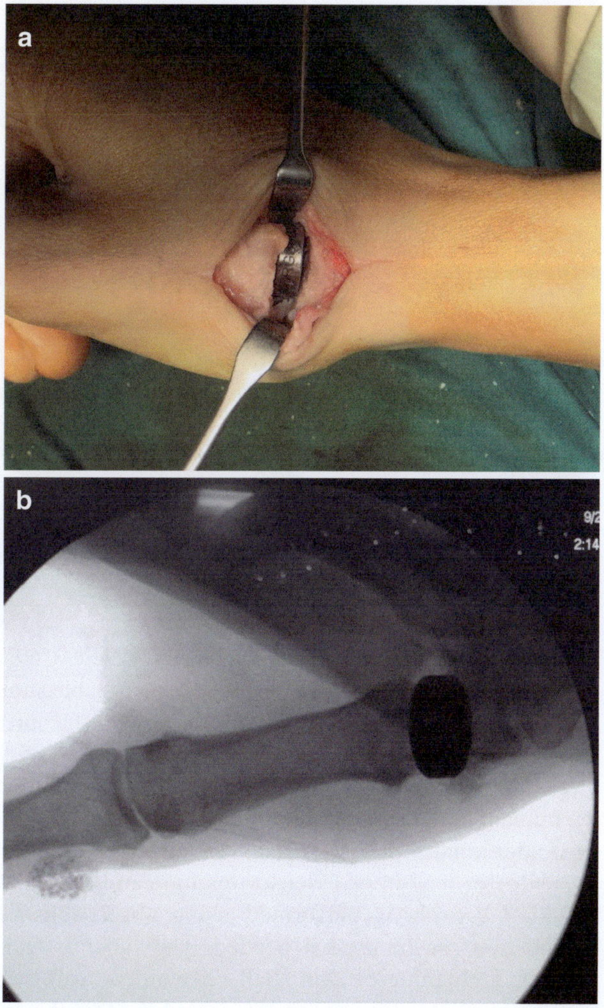

Fig. 7.21 (**a**, **b**) RegJoint sizer: the spacer must be large as the first metacarpal base surface at the fluoroscan

Fig. 7.22 The implant is positioned in the space between first metacarpal bone and trapezium, and the capsule is sutured

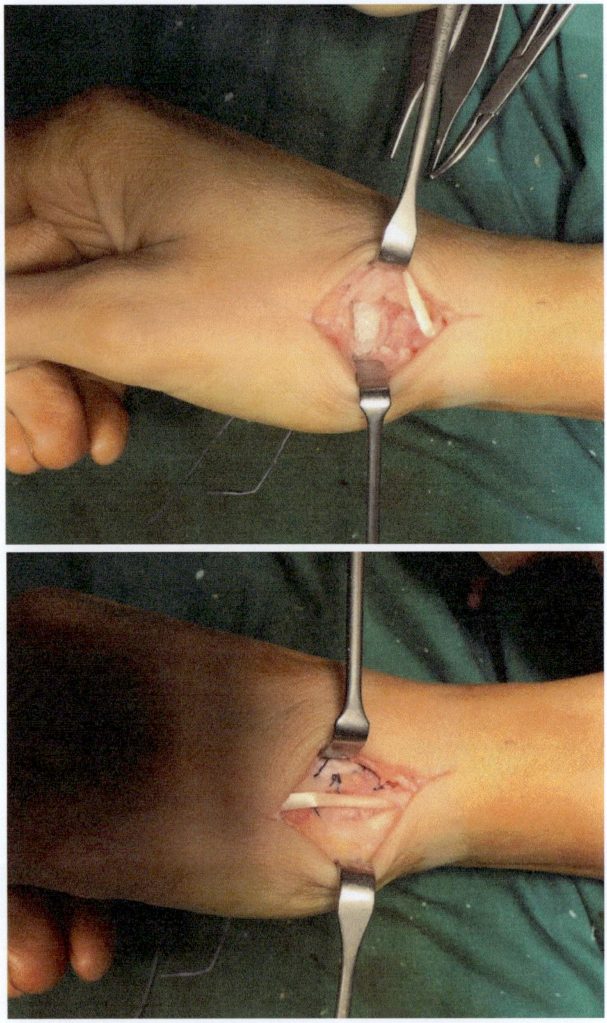

RegJoint™ is fixed with transosseous resorbable sutures (e.g. PDS 2-0); the scaffold can be fixed into the joint capsule or with the surrounded flexor carpi radialis tendon. Alternatively, RegJoint™ can also be fixed with a temporary K-wire going through the first metacarpal (or the whole thumb) to the resected joint line piercing the implant and trapezium up to the carpals.

If additional support is needed, a tendon interposition from flexor carpi radialis, abductor tendon or extensor tendon can be used. A careful reconstruction of the joint capsule is performed using absorbable suture material (Fig. 7.22). Duplication can be used if needed. The subcutis and skin are closed in routine manner. Tightening of skin shall be avoided. Soft bandage and a gipsy cast or a temporary plaster for immobilization of the thumb can be used. On the second or

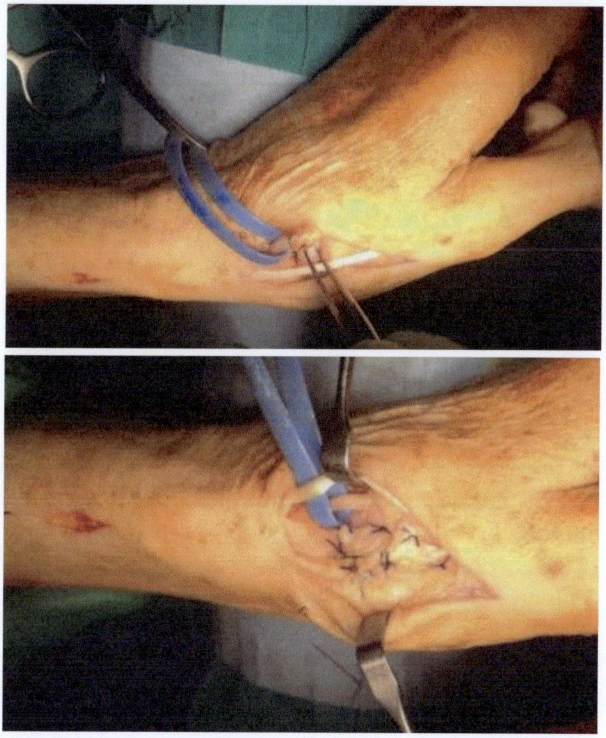

Fig. 7.23 In case of trapeziectomy, the spacer is inserted alone or in association with a LRTI, in this case the ALP has been used; the spacer is fixed to the ALP using absorbable sutures

third postoperative day, the plaster is removed, and an orthose (e.g. hexalite, neoprene or thermoplastic material) can be applied for 4–6 weeks. External K-wire, if used, is removed after 3–4 weeks. Range-of-motion exercises are allowed after 4–6 weeks using a special training splint. After 6 weeks, a functional abduction splint is applied if needed. Rehabilitation and physiotherapy are planned individually for each patient.

This scaffold is promising and is very versatile; it can be used in case of hemi-trapeziectomy or instead of LRTI in case of total trapeziectomy; if the surgeon is worried about stability in case of a bad quality of capsule tissue, the scaffold can be fixed using ABDL, passing through the implant and inserting it at the first metacarpal base (Fig. 7.23).

If, in early OA stages, in presence of a good trapezium bone stock, a hemi-trapeziectomy is performed, it's important to evaluate accurately the space between trapezium and the base of the first metacarpal to avoid a subluxation of the implant, which is caused by a too tight arthroplasty.

Another important option is the CMC arthrodesis: in patients that are younger than 60 years and hard worker and have restricted ROM and stage III OA but are associated to an STT joint safe and to a trapezial good bone stock, this is a valid solution; it permits to recover good strength and complete pain relief, and even if there's a lost of movement, patients are satisfied.

7.3.4 Surgical Technique

An informed consent was taken, and dry arthroscopy was performed under regional anaesthesia, with the patient in supine position and pneumatic tourniquet, preset to 250 mmHg. A single finger trap on the thumb was used to suspend the extremity vertically with the wrist in neutral and ulnar deviation, and 2–3 kg of longitudinal traction was applied. Two portals were used along the TMC joint line: one immediately radial to the abductor pollicis longus, or (1-R portal), and the other immediately ulnar to the extensor pollicis brevis, or (1-U portal) (Fig. 7.2). To estimate the angle of entry, a 20-G needle was advanced into the joint. An incision was then made with a No. 15 scalpel over each portal mark, cutting only the skin. Subcutaneous tissues were bluntly dissected, using a small haemostat. When the blunt dissection reached the TMC joint capsule, a blunt tapered trocar and its sheath were introduced. Fluoroscopic confirmation of trocar placement within the TMC joint was obtained. A 1.9-mm arthroscope was used, and a 2.9-mm shaver was introduced first for debridement and synovectomy; afterwards a 2.9-mm barrel abrader was introduced, and the articular surface of the trapezium and base of the first metacarpal bone were removed in a systematic manner from ulnar to radial. The resection continued until complete removal of the articular cartilage and only cancellous bone was visualized, maintaining smooth surfaces and avoiding the creation of troughs with the burr. Then the traction was eliminated to allow for better coaptation between articular surfaces of the first metacarpal bone and the trapezium, and fluoroscopic-guided percutaneous insertion of two 2.5-mm cannulated compression screws was performed in a crossing manner from the base of the first metacarpal bone into the trapezium (Fig. 7.3), aimed at fixing the TMC joint in wire for the cannulated screws across the joint. The duration of the intervention was 40 min.

The portals were then closed, and a thumb splint was applied. Immobilization was continued for a period of 6 weeks in the form of thermoplastic custom-made splint fixing the metacarpophalangeal joint and the wrist (Fig. 7.5), and routine postoperative radiographs were obtained at 6 weeks. At 6 weeks, the DASH score improved from 61 before surgery to 10 after surgery. The preoperative VAS improved from 8 to 2, and the pinch grip strength improved from 2.5 to 8.8 kg. The preoperative grip strength was 21 kg compared to 35 kg postoperatively. Radiologically, fusion of TMC joint was obtained (Fig. 7.6), and the patient was satisfied to resume training and competition. At last clinical follow-up at 1 year (Fig. 7.7), the DASH score was 2, VAS became 0, and the pinch and hand grip strength was 10 and 38 kg, respectively, which represented 98.65% of the contralateral side.

The arthroscopic approach permits to evaluate cartilage erosion and to remove cartilage completely, avoiding one of the most important cause of non-union [38].

7.3.5 Open Surgical Technique

The approach to the joint is dorsal; care was taken to sensory branch of radial nerve and the lateral antebrachial cutaneous nerve; the radial artery was identified and protected; a longitudinal traction is applied to the joint to expose and remove the articular surface using an oscillating saw until cancellous bone is exposed and the two surfaces are parallel to obtain a full contact in the correct position for fusion. The amount of resection is minimal. The position of the arthrodesis is such that the distal phalanx of the thumb, rested on the middle phalanx of the second finger of a fully clenched fist, as described by Leach and Bolton [39] to prevent hyperextension of the metacarpophalangeal joint, can be used a bone graft. The fluoroscopic control shows a correct position of the surfaces, and a good contact fixation can be performed by K-wire or by an L-shaped locking plate and screws.

If a plate and screws are used, Abe and Tokunaga suggested early active mobilization avoiding any cast postoperatively [40].

Literature referred about complications caused by mispositioned plates and screws, delay in union or non-union, limited ROM and arthritis of near joint and the criticism of limited ROM, on average abduction and adduction are reduced by 72% and flexion, and extension are reduced by 61%. Limited motion is compensated by increased motion at the scaphotrapezial and metacarpophalangeal joints. This condition does not affect patient satisfaction [40].

In case of patient younger than 70 years, non-hard worker, limited ROM, stage III or IV of OA and STT joint involved, a surgical option could be total trapeziectomy and spacer interposition.

Trapeziectomy combined to ligamentoplasty is the simpler technique, the one that many authors consider the best solution; but this technique has the disadvantage that gives a discontinuity to the first osseous column, and the reduction of the space between the first metacarpal and the scaphoid causes the hypertension of the metacarpophalangeal joint and the reduction of the strength. A solution could be the interposition of a spacer in pyrocarbon combined to a ligamentoplasty [41, 42].

7.3.5.1 Surgical Technique

The surgery was performed under local anaesthesia and tourniquet. By way of first Gedda-Moberg [43], a longitudinal tenotomy of the abductor pollicis longus was performed to expose the joint capsule. The capsule was incised longitudinally, and the base of the first metacarpal bone was exposed and resected with an oscillating saw. Osteophytes, including medial, have been resected. Trapeziectomy was carried out step by step, ideally in one piece with a lag, preserving the tendon of the flexor carpi radialis (FCR); the trapezoid was prepared using a burr to accommodate the implant Pi21.

The bone tunnel for the passage of the ligament was carried out to the motor in the base of the first metacarpal bone, parallel to the nail bed. The synthetic wire or the tendon was passed around the FCR to form a head node lark, as distally as possible, and the end of the ligament was passed in the FCR to avoid sliding on the tendon. Then, the first bone passage was made in the medial opening of the extra bone metacarpal endomedullary where the needle was recovered. It was then pressed in the FCR, always distally. The second passage of the ligamentoplasty was then directed by the side port of the metacarpal always extra in endomedullary. Both strands were then knotted; the implant Pi2 was introduced after realizing the ligament. The capsule was then sutured in overcoat to avoid dislocation of the implant.

The skin was sutured with interrupted sutures. Patients were immobilized for 5 weeks with a splint commissure, leaving free the wrist.

Even if the space between scaphoid and first metacarpal bone is preserved, literature does not refer about better results; the only parameter that benefits of this condition is the reduction of hyperextension of metacarpophalangeal joint; but in 30% of cases, the implant was sub-dislocated or dislocated causing an important discomfort.

There's no evidence that the implant interposition gives better results than simple trapeziectomy combined to ligamentoplasty.

7.4 Surgical Approaches: Arthroplasty Without Interposition Implants

In patients affected by rizoarthritis older than 65–70 years, limited ROM, low demanding the best solution is trapeziectomy and ligamentoplasty.

Starting from 1973 several authors described different ways to perform the trapeziectomy: simple, associated to ligamentoplasty, combined to ligamentoplasty and tendon interposition, using different tendon or synthetic ligament to perform the ligamentoplasty and interposition.

Gervis in 1949 [1] described a simple trapeziectomy; ligamentoplasty and interposition were thought to avoid the collapse of the space between scaphoid and first metacarpal bone.

Surgical technique: The limb is exsanguinated by application of an Esmarch bandage. A pneumatic tourniquet is placed on the upper arm and is inflated to 250 mmHg. The incisions (a dorsoradial incision, about 7 cm long, S-shaped, centred over the trapeziometacarpal joint, and four incisions, about 1.5 cm each, 4 cm apart from each other, longitudinally placed over the course of the tendon of flexor carpi radialis) are carefully delineated with a marker pen. After skin incision, the radial artery and vein and the dorsal cutaneous nerves are carefully retracted.

The trapeziometacarpal joint is exposed by opening its capsule. The articular surface of the base of the first metacarpal is removed with a power saw.

The trapezium is excised piecemeal, taking care not to damage the underlying tendon of flexor carpi radialis.

The radial one-third to one-half of the flexor carpi radialis tendon is harvested after longitudinal splitting through the multiple longitudinal incisions after having been split over a distance of 10–12 cm.

The tendon strip is developed distally to the base of the second metacarpal, taking care not to detach it distally. The skin wounds are sutured with interrupted ethylon.

A hole is drilled in the radial cortex of the base of the first metacarpal passing proximally to the centre of the base of the metacarpal, perpendicular to the plane of the finger nail.

Accurate spatial positioning of the thumb in relation to the index finger is necessary. The flexor carpi radialis tendon strip is passed through the hole at the base of the first metacarpal in an ulnar-to-radial direction (drill 2.5 mm).

The position is held by percutaneous fixation with a K-wire (1.5 mm) through the lateral cortex of the first metacarpal passing proximal and medially into the carpus while holding the thumb in a position of opposition and taking care not to lengthen the thumb.

The tendon is sutured back onto itself at the base of the metacarpal, thus reconstructing the palmar ligament between the bases of the second and first metacarpals and preventing proximal and dorsal migration of the thumb metacarpal.

The remaining part of the tendon is folded onto itself and packed in the space previously occupied by the trapezium. In this way, the radial portion of the flexor carpi radialis tendon acts as a spacer, preventing proximal migration of the first metacarpal. The skin is sutured with interrupted 5-0 ethylon. This surgical procedure is the original one described by Maffulli in 1997; the only difference in performing the procedure from the original Burton's technique was making longitudinal instead of transverse incisions over the course of the tendon of flexor carpi radialis and of not suturing the tendon of flexor carpi radialis onto itself in the space produced by excising the trapezium.

In postoperative period, a cast was applied for 6 weeks, and the K-wire was removed after an X-ray check after 6 weeks. The authors referred about good results in pain relief, recovered ROM and patient's satisfaction [44].

Weilby in 1988 described this surgical procedure to take care of basal thumb arthritis [45]: surgeries were performed under tourniquet control. First, an incision was made along the radial border of the metacarpal of the thumb, after which the trapezium was removed. Great care was taken to avoid injury to the superficial radial nerve. A tendon strip about 10 cm in length and consisting of approximately one-third of the width of the FCR tendon was dissected and tunnelled to its insertion on the second metacarpal. This tendon graft was then intertwined in a figure-of-eight fashion (at least twice) around the abductor pollicis longus tendon and the rest of the FCR tendon, pulling those tendons together into the space created after excision of the trapezium bone. The figure of eight was locked by a non-absorbable 3-0 suture. The remaining tendon graft was wrapped upon itself as described by Carrol in 1987 [46] and was interposed in the space left after the removal of the trapezium and pushed between the base of the first and second metacarpals. The joint capsule was closed, but K-wires were not inserted to stabilize the thumb. The thumb was immobilized in a spica cast for 4 weeks, after which the cast was replaced with a removable protective splint and physiotherapy was started by a hand therapist. Vermeulen concluded that the Weilby procedure is a reliable alternative to treat primary thumb carpometacarpal osteoarthritis without requiring bone tunnel creation. It achieves pain relief, stability, mobility and strength. The objective and subjective outcomes of this study compare favourably with those of earlier reports of the Weilby procedure and are similar to the published results of the more commonly performed Burton-Pellegrini technique.

A different way to perform this kind of arthroplasty is the stripping of the most volar part of abductor longus pollicis (ALP) to its insertion on the basal first metacarpal; the stripped tendon is passed under FCR tendon and then fixed to the dorsal side of the first metacarpal bone; the tendon in excess is made as an anchovy and positioned in the space between scaphoid and first metacarpal bone (Fig. 7.24).

Arthroplasty according to Ceruso also involves the use of the long abductor tendon of the thumb instead of the radial flexor of the carpus, once the trapezius is removed, the tendon band is taken with the dorsal component of the ALP tendon, disentangling it proximally. The Author then proceeds to its suspension with passing through and around the FRC by a double turn passed first through an eyelet made in the most distal portion of the FRC and a second time around the entire tendon. The bandage is then stabilized with intracapsular passage and suture to the joint capsule with a non-resorbable suture thread. Post-operative immobilization includes a plaster with included first finger and metacarpus in slight abduction for 4 weeks followed by 6 others with only night splitting [47]. The ligamentoplasty developed by Francesco Brunelli is based on the anchoring of the fly band of the ALP tendon to the first dorsal intermetacarpal ligament, in order to obtain a suspension arthroplasty that does not include sutures on other tendons or skeletal tunneling. The technique foresees the use of the ALP volar band to create a suspension ligament which constitutes a "hammock" for the first metacarpal bone, which is anchored to the fascia on the radial side and to the first dorsal intermetacarpal ligament on the ulnar side [48].

A different solution without ligamentoplasty and tendon interposition was suggested by Kuhns in 2003 [49]: the haematoma distraction (HAD). The surgical procedure consisted of a curved dorsal radial incision over the trapezium, multiple longitudinal fractionations of the trapezium with an osteotome and piecemeal excision of the entire trapezium using a combination of sharp dissection and rongeur avulsion. No ligament reconstruction or tendon interposition was used. With the thumb in wide palmar abduction, slight opposition and distraction until firm resistance was encountered, a single 1.6-mm K-wire was passed from the first metacarpal base in a proximal-dorsal-ulnar direction until it engaged securely in either the base of the second metacarpal or in the trapezoid. The trailing end of the K-wire was left exposed at the insertion site. All procedures were performed with Bier block regional anaesthesia. Surgical time for the haematoma and distraction arthroplasty alone was 35 min (range, 25–47 min).

A short-arm thumb spica splint immobilized the reconstruction for the first 10 days. After suture removal, a short-arm thumb spica cast was applied for 5 weeks after surgery. In the HDA the K-wire holds the first metacarpal in a distracted position. This allows the largest possible space for haematoma and eventual fibrosis to develop during the postoperative immobilization. The X-ray also shows the first and second metacarpal bases in close proximity. This allows the fibrous tissue that naturally forms during the 5 weeks of K-wire immobilization to support the thumb metacarpal base in a manner quite similar to the native or formally reconstructed anterior oblique ligament. Meals, in 2003, referred about results that support the concept that K-wire immobilization in a slightly overcorrected position without formal interposition or ligament reconstruction allows for restoration of a stable,

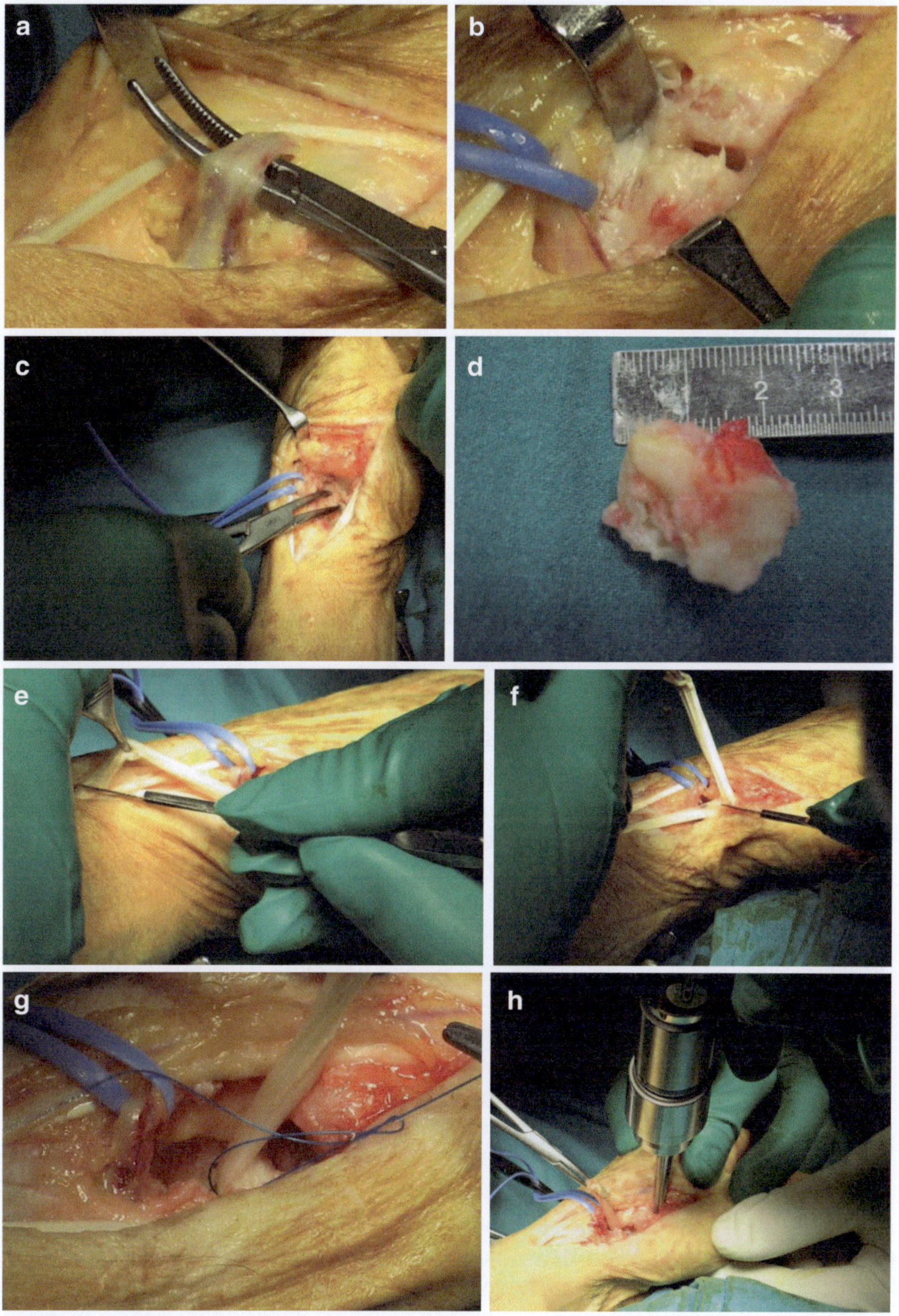

Fig. 7.24 Weilby modified procedure: (**a**) radial artery; (**b**) capsulotomy; (**c**, **d**) trapeziectomy; (**e**, **f**) preparation of ALP; (**g**, **h**) tenosuspension. The ALP is passed under FCR tendon, sutured to FCR tendon using nylon 3/0 and fixed to the dorsal side of first metacarpal bone using a mini anchor; the tendon in excess is shaped as an anchovy and positioned in the space between scaphoid and first metacarpal bone

pain-free thumb that has superior strength and motion compared with the more complicated interventions [45]. However, the longevity of HDA and its durability over time are unknown. Potential for increased proximal migration in the HDA group exists and is a concern that may eventually lead to a weaker thumb and pain from abutment on the distal scaphoid, but the LRTI arthroplasty is a considerably longer and more complex surgery than the HAD [50], and literature considers the space between scaphoid and first metacarpal bone not so crucial for good clinical results [13].

An alternative option to perform LRTI in case of rizoarthritis and STT arthritis is to use the APL instead of FCR. Thompson is the first author who described this technique in 1886 [6]. Kochevar [9] did a revision of this procedure in 2011 to a group of patients with a follow-up of 5.5 years. Sammer described the technique in 2010 [51]: The surgery is generally performed under regional anaesthesia. The hand and forearm are exsanguinated, and the tourniquet is inflated to 250 mmHg. An incision is made over the radial aspect of the thumb basal joint and carried down through skin and subcutaneous tissue. Branches of the radial sensory nerve are identified and protected. The first extensor compartment is sharply opened along its dorsal aspect. Often there is a separate sub-sheath for the extensor pollicis brevis (EPB) and multiple slips of the abductor pollicis longus (APL). The interval between the APL and EPB is opened. The tendons are retracted to each side, and the radial artery is identified, dissected free, and retracted proximally. The trapeziometacarpal and scaphotrapezial (ST) joints are opened and inspected. If the ST joint appears uninvolved; a partial trapeziectomy with preservation of the ST joint may be performed. Otherwise, a complete trapeziectomy should be performed. One of the dorsal slips of the APL is then detached as proximally as possible in the forearm through the existing incision. It is retrieved into the wound and then passed under the EPB and radial artery in a dorsal and ulnar direction towards the extensor carpi radialis longus (ECRL). The APL is then passed through the ECRL as distally as possible, turned back along itself, pulled tight and sutured to itself with interrupted 2-0 braided suture, thus stabilizing the carpometacarpal joint. It is important at this step to confirm the stability of the reconstruction by attempting to translate to thumb metacarpal from side to side, as one would in performing the carpometacarpal grind test. No motion should be possible. If some laxity is noted, the braided sutures are removed, the APL slip is pulled tighter and the sutures are placed again. Once the surgeon is satisfied with the stability of the reconstruction, the tourniquet is deflated, haemostasis is achieved, and the skin incision is closed. A sterile dressing and thumb spica splint are applied. Postoperatively, the patient begins gentle active finger range of motion immediately. The plaster splint is removed and replaced with a short-arm thumb spica cast within a few days of surgery. The cast and sutures are removed in 10–14 days. The patient is placed in a removable thermoplastic forearm-based thumb spica splint and instructed in gentle active thumb range of motion and light functional activities. At 6 weeks postoperatively, the patient begins to wean off of the splint and to increase activity level as comfort permits. Usually patients are able to return to full activity within 3–4 months [50]. This technique is a useful addition to the hand surgeon's armamentarium for the treatment of thumb basal joint arthritis. Its advantages are that it is straightforward to perform and teach, it does not require additional forearm incisions or sacrifice of the FCR and it creates a suspensionplasty without the need for bone tunnels. Even if the loss of trapezial space is not correlated to unsatisfying clinical results, some type of interposition and ligamentoplasty may improve stability and decrease the possibility of scapho-metacarpal impingement.

Singer described a similar procedure using APL in 2015: he used a Wagner approach to expose the TMC joint; the capsule was longitudinally incised and the trapezium resected by enucleation after complete release of attachment inside the capsule or piecemeal removal using a rongeur, taking care not to damage FCR; the APL is identified; and the dorsal part of it is dissected and cut 3.5 cm from the insertion; this slip is then looped around FCR from behind to forward two or three times to maintain traction on the thumb and to preserve trapezial space height. This rolled loop occupied the trapezium space, acting as a spacer maintaining height, avoiding laxity and supporting the base of first metacarpal as a hammock. Postoperatively a cast is used for 3 weeks.

The LRTI by Burton and Pellegrini [52], performed to reconstruct the anterior oblique ligament, has been associated with weakness in wrist flexion and torsion; that's why different authors look for a different procedure. Trapeziectomy and ligamentoplasty using APL, avoiding to perform bone tunnel, in Singer's opinion are good solutions to obtain pain relief, good ROM and stability and to preserve trapezial height, with an average surgical time of half an hour.

Kinematic analysis of the thumb CMC joint in different surgical treatment demonstrated that when the trapezium is removed, an empty space between scaphoid and trapezium is created and the centre of rotation of the thumb is shifted; in adjunct the lack of articular congruity enables the metacarpal to pivot around a point closer to its base and away from the normal centre of rotation. Thompson reconstruction provides structural support similar to that of the intact joint, but the restraint of the ligament reconstruction may increase the overall joint stiffness. The Weilby procedure reduced the effective radius of motion but maintained the work area compared to the intact joint. The procedure is effective in anchoring the base of the thumb metacarpal, but it allows a big range of motion; the LRTI procedure provided a radius of joint motion and an articular area similar to those of the intact joint. The soft tissue interposition was beneficial for maintaining the radius of joint motion [53].

In the case of severe disability, hyperlassity, between I and II metacarpal (rare in the elderly patient) the technique described by Brunelli could be a good solution [54] this procedure involves the use of the ALP which, passed through the I and II metacarpal bone, reconstructs the intermetacarpal ligament restoring stability and connection to the two metacarpal, supporting also the first metacarpal bone. The same concept can be done in the modern way with the use of non-organic materials (tight rope—Arthrex).

In literature although many techniques have been described to restore motion and strength and to relieve pain in case of basal thumb osteoarthritis, none is definitely superior to the others [55–57]. The big question about the importance of maintaining the trapezial space in recovering function and strength is still open, even if it seems clinical results are not correlated to this.

But even if it's possible to give different indications in different kinds of patients, considering ages, daily living activities, kind of job, OA stages, STT arthritis and trapezium bone stock, but even if we are able to give different indications considering these factors and we can choose to remove partially or completely the trapezium, to perform a LRTI or to interpose an implant technique, there are so many that remains open to the question about which one in any different stage is the best one.

References

1. Gervis WH (1949) Excision of the trapezium for osteoarthritis of the trapezial-metacarpal joint. J Bone Joint Surg Br 31:537–250
2. Froimson AI (1970) Tendon arthroplasty of the trapeziometacarpal joint. Clin Orthop 70:191–199
3. Peimer CA, Medige J, Eckert BS, Wright JR, Howard CS (1986) Reactive synovities after silicon arthroplasty. J Hand Surg Am 11:624–638
4. Tomaino MM, Pellegrini VD Jr, Burton RI (1995) Arthroplasty of the basal joint of the thumb. Long term follow up after ligament reconstruction with tendon interposition. J Bone Joint Surg Am 77:346–355
5. Illarramendi AA, Borretto JG, Gallucci GL, DeCarli P (2006) Trapeziecotmy and intermetacarpal ligament reconstruction with the extensor carpi radialis longus for osteoarthritis of the trapeziometacarpal joint: surgical technique and long term result. J Hand Surg Am 31:1315–1321
6. Thompson JS (1986) Surgical treatment of trapeziometacarpal arthrosis. Adv Orthop Surg 10:105–120
7. Thompson JS (1989) Complication and salvage of trapeziometacarpal arthroplasties. Am Acad Orthop Surg 38:3–13
8. Brunelli L, Monini L, Brunelli F (1989) Stabilization of trapeziometacarpal joint. J Hand Surg Br 14:209–212
9. Kochevar AJ, Adhams CN, Adham MN, Angel MF, Walkinshaw MD (2011) Thumb basal joint arthroplasty using abductor pollicis longus tendon: an average 5.5-year follow up. J Hand Surg Am 36:1326–1332
10. Soejima O, Hanamura T, Kikuta T, Lida H, Nito M (2006) Suspensionplasty with the abductor pollicis longus tendon for osteoarthritis in the carpometacarpal joint of the thumb. J Hand Surg Am 31:425–428
11. Belcher HJ, Nicholl JE (2000) A comparison of trapeziectomy with and without ligament reconstruction and tendon interposition. J Hand Surg Br 25:350–356
12. Downing ND, Davis TR (2001) Trapezial space height after trapeziectomy: mechanism of formation and benefit. J Hand Surg Am 26:862–868
13. Luria S, Waitayawinyu T, Nemechek N, Huber P, Tencer A, Trumble T (2007) Biomechanic analysis of trapeziectpmy ligament reconstruction with tendon interposition and tie-it trapezium implant arthropalsty fot thumb carpometacrpal arthritis: a cadver stady. J Hand Surg AM 32:697–706
14. Vermeulen GM, Slijper H, Feitz R, Hovius SER, Moojen TM, Selles RW (2011) Surgical management of primary thumb carpometacrpal ostheoarthritis: a systematic review. J Hand Surg Am 36:157–169
15. Martou G, Veltri K, Thomas A (2004) Surgical treatment of osteoarthritis of the carpo metacarpal joint of the thumb: a systematic review. Plast Reconstr Surg 114:421–432
16. Wajon A, Ada L, Edmund I (2005) Surgery for thumb (trapeziometacarpal joint) osteoarthritis. Cochrane Database Syst Rev (4):CD004631
17. Wajon A, Carr E, Edmund I, Ada L (2009) Surgery for thumb (trapeziometacarpal joint) osteoarthritis. Cochrane Database Syst Rev (2):CD004631

18. Taylor EJ, Desari K, D'Arcy JC, Bonnici AV (2005) A comparison of fusion, trapeziectomy and silastic replacement for the treatment of osteoarthritis of the trapeziometacarpal joint. J Hand Surg Br 30:45–49
19. Garcia-Mas R, Sole Molinas X (2005) Partial trapeziectomy with ligament reconstruction–tendon interposition and silastic replacement for the treatment of osteoarthritis of the trapeziometacarpal joint. J Hand Surg Br 30:45–49
20. Forseth MJ, Stern PJ (2003) Complication of trapeziometacarpal Arthrodesis using plate and screws fixation. J Hand Surg Am 28:342–345
21. Ulrich-Vinther M, Puggard H, Lange B (2008) Prospective 1-year follow up study comparing joint prosthesis with tendon interposition arhroplasty in treatment of trapeziometacarpal osteoarthritis. J Hand Surg Am 33:1369–1377
22. Wilson JN (1973) Basal osteotomy of the first metacarpal in the treatment of arthritis of the carpometacarpal joint of the thumb. Br J Surg 60:854–858
23. Eaton RG, Littler JW (1973) Ligament reconstruction for the painful thumb carpometacrpal joint. J Bone Joint Surg Am 55:1655–1666
24. Raven EEJ, Kerkhoffs GMMJ, Rutten S, Marsman AJW, Mrti RK, Albers GHR (2007) Long term results of surgical intervention for osteoarthritis of the trapezio metacarpal joint. Int Orthop (SICOT) 31:547–554
25. Dacatra U, Odella S, Torretta F (2008) Artrosi trapezio-metacarpale: inquadramento clinico e impostazione di un algoritmo di trattamento. Archivio di ortopedia e traumatologia 118(4):19
26. Scroder J, Kertkhoffs GMMJ, Voerman HJ (2002) Surgical treatment of the thumb: comparison between resection-interposition arthroplasty and trapezio-metacarpal arthrodesis. Arch Orthop Trauma Surg 122:35–38
27. Woodward JF, Heller JB, Jones e F (2013) Pyrocarbon implant hemiarthroplasty for trapeziometacarpal arthritis. Tech Hand Up Extrem Surg 17:7–12
28. Pérez-Úbeda M-J, Garćia-López A, Marco Martinez F, Junyent Vilanova E, Molina Martos M, López-Duran Stern L (2003) Results of the cemented SR trapeziometacarpal prosthesis in the treatment of thumb carpometacarpal osteoarthritis. J Hand Surg Am 28:917–925
29. Nicholas RM, Calderwood JW (1992) De la caffinière arthroplasty for basal thumb joint osteoarthritis. J Bone Joint Surg Br 74:309–312
30. Glickel SZ (2001) Clinical assessment of the thumb trapeziometacarpal joint. Hand Clin 17:185–195
31. Linscheid RL (2000) Implant arthroplasty of the hand: retrospec- tive and prospective considerations. J Hand Surg Am 25:796–816
32. Badia A (2008) Total joint arthroplasty for the arthritic thumb carpometacarpal joint. Am J Orthop 37(8 suppl):4–7
33. Cook T, Kester J (1989) Wear characteristics of the canine acetabulum against different femoral prosthesis. J Bone Joint Surg Br 71(2):189–197
34. Igoe D, Middelton C, Hammert W (2014) Evolution of basal joint arthroplasty and technology in hand surgery. J Hand Ther 27:115–121
35. Bellemère P, Gaisne E, Loubersac T, Ardouin L, Collon S, Maes C (2011) L'implant Pyrocardan: interposition libre en pyrocarbone pour resurfaçage de l'articulation trapézométacarpienne. Chirurgie de la main 30:S28–S35
36. Stabler D (2011) Pyrodisk trapezium replacement. In: Abstract book Australian Hand Surgery Society Annual Meeting, Bunker Bay, Australia
37. Odella S, Querenghi AM, Sartore R, DeFelice A, Dacatra U (2014) Trapeziometacarpal osteoarthritis: pyrocarbon interposition implants. Joints 2(4):154–158
38. Mohamed A, Yousef A, Pegoli L (2013) Arthroscopic-assisted arthrodesis of the trapeziometacarpal joint. Tech Hand Up Extrem Surg 17:116–119
39. Leach RE, Bolton PE (1968) Arthritis of the caprometacarpal joint of the thumb: results of arthrodesis. J Bone Joint Surg Am 50:1171–1177
40. Abe Y, Tokunaga S (2015) Surgical technique and clinical results for trapeziometacarpal arthrodesis using locking plate fixation in women aged 50 years or older. Plast Reconstr Surg 136:521–528

41. Stussi JD, Dap F, Merle M (2000) Étude rétrospective de 69 rhizarthroses primitives opérées par trapézectomie totale suivie dans 34 cas de tendino-plastie d'interposition et dans 35 cas de suspensioplastie. Chir Main 19:116–127
42. Camus E, Farez E, Rtaimate M, Millot F, Bouretz JC (2000) Traitement chirurgical de la rhizarthrose par trapézectomie-interposition-ligamento-plastie. Chir Main 19:36–43
43. Gedda KO, Moberg E (1953) Open reduction and osteosynthesis of the so-called Bennett's fracture in the carpo-metacarpal joint of the thumb. Acta Orthop Scand 22:249–257
44. Maffulli N, Ierwin I, Buchan CR (1997) Modified Burton and pellegrini procedure for trapezium excision, ligament reconstruction and interposition arthroplasty of the tendon of flexor carpi radialis. Oper Orthop Traumatol 9:69–79
45. Weilby A (1988) Tendon interposition arthroplasty of the first carpo-metacarpal joint. J Hand Surg Br 13:421–425
46. Carroll RE (1987) Arthrodesis of the carpometacarpal joint of the thumb. A review of patients with a long postoperative period. Clin Orthop Relat Res 220:106–110
47. Caruso. M. Innocenti M, Angelini R, Laoui G, Bufalini C. L'artrosi del primo raggio digitale. riv Chir Mano 1991;28:67–75
48. Brunelli G, Monini L, Brunelli F. Stabilizzazione della trapeziometacarpale nella rizoartrosi G.I.O.T. 1988;16;371–376
49. Kuhns CA, Emerson ET, Meals RA (2003) Hematoma and distraction arthroplasty for thumb basal joint osteoarthritis: a prospective, single-surgeon study including outcomes measures. J Hand Surg Am 28(3):381–389
50. Sandvall BK, Cameron TE, Netscher DT, Epstein MJ, Staines KG, Petersen NJ (2010) Basal joint osteoarthritis of the thumb: ligament reconstruction and tendon interposition versus hematoma distraction arthroplasty. J Hand Surg Am 35:1968–1975
51. Sammer DM, Amadio PC (2010) Description and outcomes of a new technique for thumb basal joint arthroplasty. J Hand Surg Am 35:1198–1205
52. Burton R, Pellegrini V (1986) Surgical management for basal thumb osteoarthritis: part II. Ligament reconstruction with tendon interposition arthroplasty. J Hand Surg Am 11:324–332
53. Koff MF, Shao KD, Mierisch CM, Chen M-Y, An K-N, Cooney WP III (2007) Jpint kinematics after thumb carpometacrpal joint reconstruction: an in vitro comparison of various constructs. J Hand Surg Am 32:688–696
54. Brunelli GR. Instabilità della articolazione trapeziometacarpale, rizartrosi. La Mano, manuale di chirurgia. Edi.erms. 20:337–49.
55. Colegate-Stone TJ, Garg S, Subramanian A, Mani GV (2011) Outcome analysis of trapeziectomy with and without pyrocarbon interposition to treat primary arthrosis of the trapeziometacarpal joint. Hand Surg 16:49–54
56. Szalay G, Schleicher I, Alt V, Pavlidis T, Schnettler R (2011) Operativetreatment of rhizarthritis: comparison of ligament reconstruction according to Epping with trapeziectomy and interposition of pyrocarbon spacers as replacement of the trapezium. Orthopade 40:237–246
57. Cheval D, Sauleau V, Moineau G, Le Jacques B, Le Nen D (2013) Trapézectomie totale et ligamentoplastie de suspension: une interposition par un implant Pi2[1] en pyrocarbone a-t-elle un intérêt? Chirurgie de la main 32:169–175

Conclusions

Trapezio-metacarpal arthritis is a common affection in female population over 50 years, in menopausal age with a radiographic prevalence of 36%; in the fifth and sixth decade in male population, the X-ray prevalence is 13%; in population over 80 years old, 91% of people are affected by thumb osteoarthritis; this condition causes hand dysfunction in some patients [1–5].

Probably, it is a multifactorial condition; ligaments, hormones, anatomical condition, kind of hand activity are important elements to be considered; the pathophysiology of this disease is still controversial; for many years, the anterior oblique ligament failure has been considered the most responsible for the thumb osteoarthritis. Pellegrini described the ligamentous laxity theory that demonstrated the correlation between anterior volar beak ligament and chondral wear [6, 7].

Other authors stressed the importance of dorsal ligaments; they noticed that the subluxation never happens in case of dorso-radial ligaments intact [8, 9].

The prevalence of thumb osteoarthritis in female population probably is caused by a different osseous morphology and by hormonal difference (increased level of relaxin and estrogen) [10–12].

It's a disabling condition in normal daily living activities; the limitation is mostly caused by the important pain.

The first therapy must be conservative, hand exercises, joint protection education like the avoidance of key and chuck pinch can be useful in reducing pain but not in function and strength recovery [13, 14].

Many different splints are available to reduce pain limiting CMC motion, in terms of design the one that limits CMC motion but not metacarpophalangeal ROM have been associate to better results [15, 16].

In case of failure of the hand joint education and splinting, nonsteroid anti-inflammatory drugs could help in reducing pain and improve hand function; even corticosteroid injection and hyaluronic acid represent a potential treatment; hyaluronic acid seems to be more effective than steroid in advanced diseases [14, 17, 18].

TMC joint arthritis is painful and disabling more in the initial stages than in advanced ones; this happens because in severe condition the range of motion is limited by the bones incongruity.

Surgical treatment is indicated only in case of unacceptable pain and a nonadequate response to conservative treatment [19].

S. Odella, *Trapeziometacarpal Joint Osteoarthritis*,
https://doi.org/10.1007/978-3-319-44336-2

Several different techniques are recognized; no one is proved to be superior to another; the surgeon has the possibility to choose the one that is more suitable for patient age and needs.

It's possible to perform surgery sparing or sacrificing trapezium [20]; in patients with a more severe degeneration, trapeziectomy could be a good choice, patients who present a Z deformity need a particular attention; in case of metacarpophalangeal hyperextension < than 30°, the result of trapeziectomy is not affected; if the hyperextension is > than 35°, a volar plate advancement or an arthrodesis is suggested; in case of a hyperextension >than 60°, an arthrodesis is indicated [21, 22].

There are several trapezium sacrificing procedures, starting from simple trapeziectomy that can be performed even in WALANT [19], or followed by temporary Kirschner stabilization in a distraction position to give time to the hematoma to be replaced by fibrous tissue (HAD); or in association with a tendon interposition or with a ligament reconstruction and tendon interposition (LRTI) using different tendons (flexor carpi radialis, abductor pollicis longus) or in association with a suture suspensionplasty. A 2015 Cochrane Review determined that there's no evidence of better results in case of association of LRTI to simple trapeziectomy [23].

The trapezium sparing procedures include different possibilities.

Carpometacarpal denervation: removing sensory endings should give pain relief and the preservation of the range of motion and strength but could occur hypertrophic scarring and hyperesthesia over the thumb [24].

In patients with an initial degeneration at 30°, metacarpal extension osteotomy could be a valid solution; this procedure increases grip and pinch strength even in a long follow-up [25].

Arthroscopy has been popularized by Berger to perform staging and treatment of early thumb osteoarthritis. Other authors described a debridement and hemitrapeziectomy in more advanced stage with or without tendon interposition [26–29]. Possible complications are cartilage damage or sensory branches injury.

In young patient high demanding arthrodesis is a good option; this procedure can be performed using Kischner wires, plate and screws, cannulated screws, tension band wire fixation, the fusion position should be 30–40° of palmar abduction, 10–20° of radial abduction, and extension to allow key pinch. The possible complication is nonunion or secondary reoperation.

Nowadays, the prosthetic arthroplasty hasn't found the gold standard, Swanson first suggested to use a silicon implant but complication rate was too high [30]. Pyrolytic carbon spacers were introduced with different design or degradable devices, or a metal ball and socket total joint arthroplasty; the purpose of these devices is to guaranty strength and relief pain but even this procedure can present complications as mobilization, subluxation or bone erosion, and consequent secondary surgery.

Recent literature reviews concluded that a myriad of different surgical techniques are possible when conservative treatment failed; the hand surgeon has to be familiar with the different techniques and choose the one adequate for every single patient [19, 20].

References

1. Armstrong AL, Hunter JB, Davis TR (1994) The prevalence of degenerative arthritis of the base of the thumb in post-menopausal women. J Hand Surg Br 19(3):340–341
2. Matullo KS, Ilyas A, Thoder JJ (2007) CMC arthroplasty of the thumb: a review. Hand (N Y) 2(4):232–239. Epub 2007 Aug 7
3. Sonne-Holm S, Jacobsen S (2006) Osteoarthritis of the first carpometacarpal joint: a study of radiology and clinical epidemiology. Results from the Copenhagen osteoarthritis study. Osteoarthritis Cartilage 14(5):496–500. Epub 2006 Mar 20
4. Sodha S, Ring D, Zurakowski D, Jupiter JB (2005) Prevalence of osteoarthrosis of the trapeziometacarpal joint. J Bone Joint Surg Am 87(12):2614–2618
5. Pellegrini VD Jr (1991) Osteoarthritis of the trapeziometacarpal joint: the pathophysiology of articular cartilage degeneration. I. Anatomy and pathology of the aging joint. J Hand Surg [Am] 16(6):967–974
6. Pellegrini VD Jr, Olcott CW, Hollenberg G (1993) Contact patterns in the trapeziometacarpal joint: the role of the palmar beak ligament. J Hand Surg [Am] 18(2):238–244
7. Strauch RJ, Behrman MJ, Rosenwasser MP (1994) Acute dislocation of the carpometacarpal joint of the thumb: an anatomic and cadaver study. J Hand Surg [Am] 19(1):93–98
8. Chenoweth BA, O'Mahony GD, Fitzgerald C, Stoner JA, O'Donoghue DL, Rayan GM (2017) Efficacy of dorsoradial capsulodesis for trapeziometacarpal joint instability: a cadaver study. J Hand Surg [Am] 42(1):e25–e31
9. Bettinger PC, Linscheid RL, Cooney WP III, An KN (2001) Trapezial tilt: a radiographic correlation with advanced trapeziometacarpal joint arthritis. J Hand Surg [Am] 26(4):692–697
10. Ladd AL, Weiss AP, Crisco JJ, Hagert E, Wolf JM, Glickel SZ, Yao J (2013) The thumb carpometacarpal joint: anatomy, hormones, and biomechanics. Instr Course Lect 62:165–179
11. Wolf JM, Scher DL, Etchill EW, Scott F, Williams AE, Delaronde S, King KB (2014) Relationship of relaxin hormone and thumb carpometacarpal joint arthritis. Clin Orthop Relat Res 472(4):1130–1137
12. Ateshian GA, Rosenwasser MP, Mow VC (1992) Curvature characteristics and congruence of the thumb carpometacarpal joint: differences between female and male joints. J Biomech 25(6):591–607
13. Bertozzi L, Valdes K, Vanti C, Negrini S, Pillastrini P, Villafañe JH (2015) Investigation of the effect of conservative interventions in thumb carpometacarpal osteoarthritis: systematic review and meta-analysis. Disabil Rehabil 37:2025–2043
14. Spaans AJ, van Minnen LP, Kon M, Schuurman AH, Schreuders AR, Vermeulen GM (2015) Conservative treatment of thumb base osteoarthritis: a systematic review. J Hand Surg [Am] 40:16–21.e6
15. Hamann N, Heidemann J, Heinrich K, Wu H, Bleuel J, Gonska C, Brüggemann GP (2014) Stabilization effectiveness and functionality of different thumb orthoses in female patients with first carpometacarpal joint osteoarthritis. Clin Biomech (Bristol, Avon) 29(10):1170–1176. Epub 2014 Sep 19
16. Vegt AE, Grond R, Grüschke JS, Boomsma MF, Emmelot CH, Dijkstra PU, Sluis CK (2017) The effect of two different orthoses on pain, hand function, patient satisfaction and preference in patients with thumb carpometacarpal osteoarthritis: a multicentre, crossover, randomised controlled trial. Bone Joint J 99-B(2):237–244
17. Lue S, Koppikar S, Shaikh K, Mahendira D, Towheed TE (2017) Systematic review of non-surgical therapies for osteoarthritis of the hand: an update. Osteoarthritis Cartilage 25(9):1379–1389. Epub 2017 Jun 15
18. Monfort J, Rotés-Sala D, Segalés N et al (2015) Comparative efficacy of intra-articular hyaluronic acid and corticoid injections in osteoarthritis of the first carpometacarpal joint: results of a 6-month single-masked randomized study. Joint Bone Spine 82:116–121
19. Weiss APC, Goodman AD (2018) Thumb basal joint arthritis. J Am Acad Orthop Surg 26:562–571

20. Gottschalk MB, Patel NN, Boden AL, Kakar S (2018) Treatment of basilar thumb arthritis. JBJS Rev 6(7):e4
21. Berger AJ, Meals RA (2015) Management of osteoarthrosis of the thumb joints. J Hand Surg [Am] 40:843–850
22. Patel TJ, Beredjiklian PK, Matzon JL (2013) Trapeziometacarpal joint arthritis. Curr Rev Musculoskelet Med 6(1):1–8
23. Wajon A, Vinycomb T, Carr E, Edmunds I, Ada L (2015) Surgery for thumb (trapeziometacarpal joint) osteoarthritis. Cochrane Database Syst Rev, CD004631
24. Arenas-Prat JM (2012) Wagner approach for first carpometacarpal joint denervation. Tech Hand Up Extrem Surg 16(2):107–109
25. Parker WL, Linscheid RL, Amadio PC (2008) Long- term outcomes of first metacarpal extension osteotomy in the treatment of carpal- metacarpal osteoarthritis. J Hand Surg [Am] 33(10):1737–1743
26. Berger RA (1997) A technique for arthroscopic evaluation of the first carpometacarpal joint. J Hand Surg [Am] 22(6):1077–1080
27. Badia A (2006) Trapeziometacarpal arthroscopy: a classification and treatment algorithm. Hand Clin 22(2):153–163
28. Menon J (1996 Oct) Arthroscopic management of trapeziometacarpal joint arthritis of the thumb. Arthroscopy 12(5):581–587
29. Earp BE, Leung AC, Blazar PE, Simmons BP (2008) Arthroscopic hemitrapeziectomy with tendon interposition for arthritis at the first carpometacarpal joint. Tech Hand Up Extrem Surg 12(1):38–42
30. Peimer CA (1987) Long-term complications of trapeziometacarpal silicone arthroplasty. Clin Orthop Relat Res (220):86–98

MIX
Papier aus verantwortungsvollen Quellen
Paper from responsible sources
FSC® C105338

If you have any concerns about our products,
you can contact us on
ProductSafety@springernature.com

In case Publisher is established outside the EU,
the EU authorized representative is:
Springer Nature Customer Service Center GmbH
Europaplatz 3, 69115 Heidelberg, Germany

Printed by Libri Plureos GmbH
in Hamburg, Germany